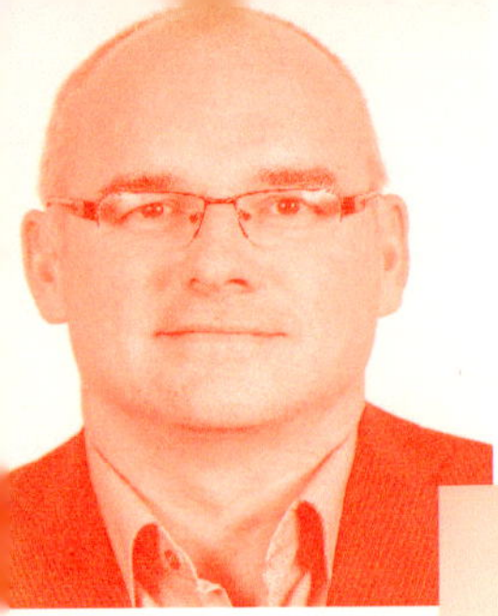
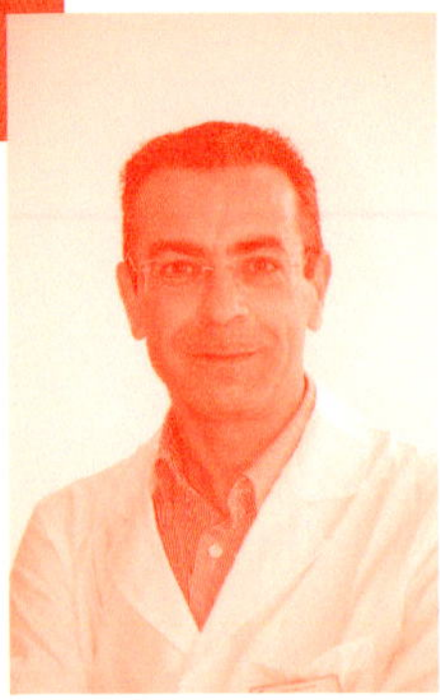
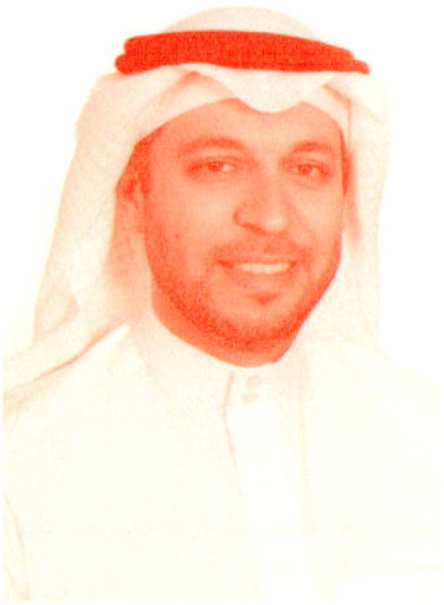
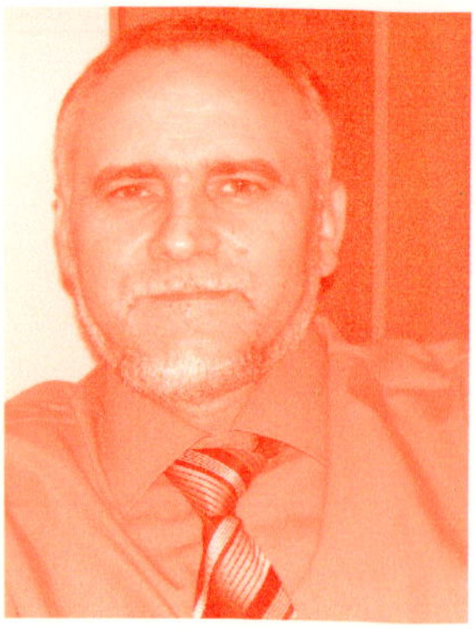
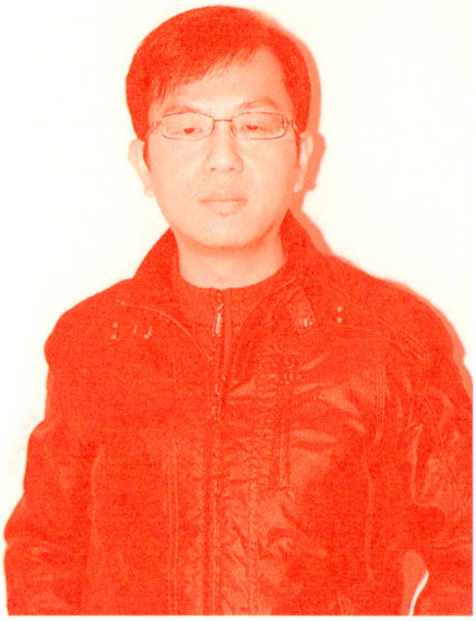
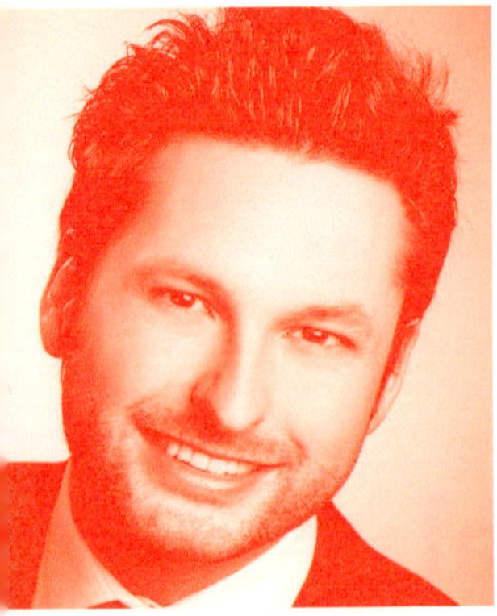
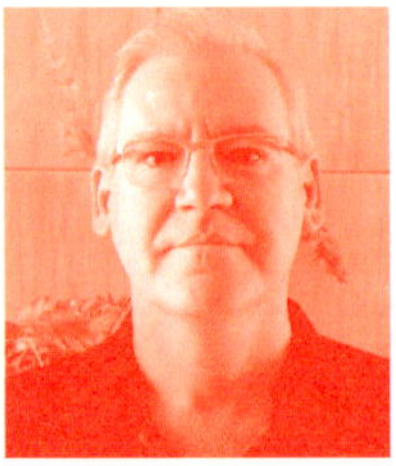

IntechOpen

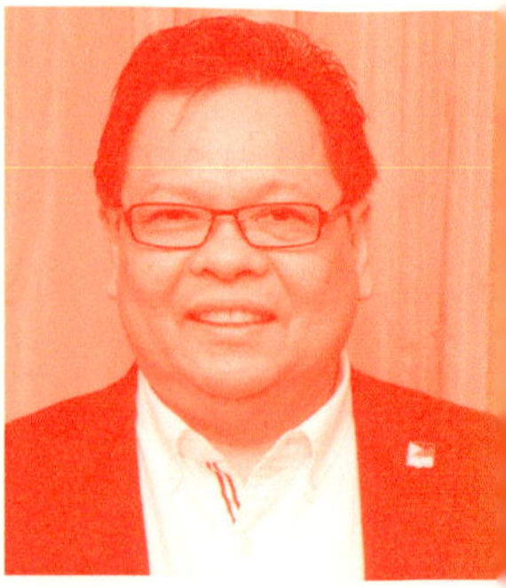
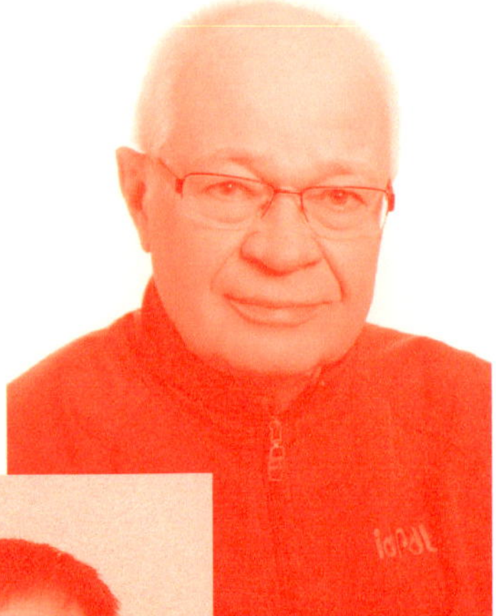
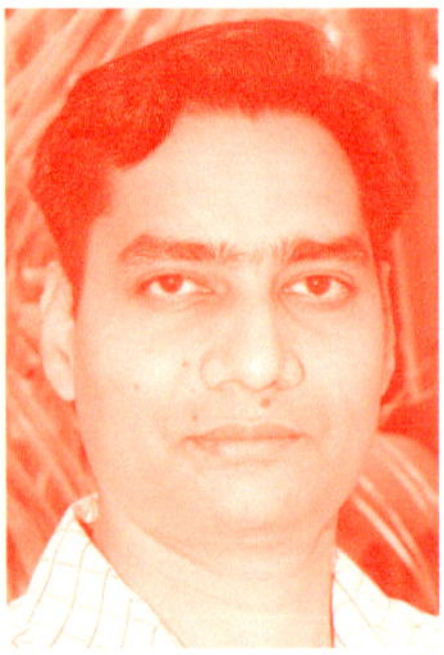
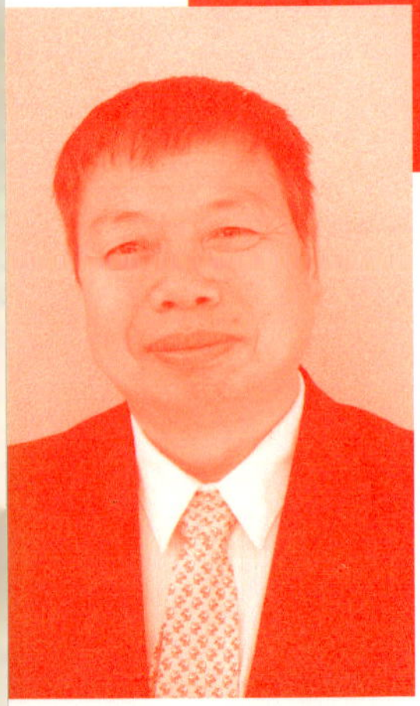
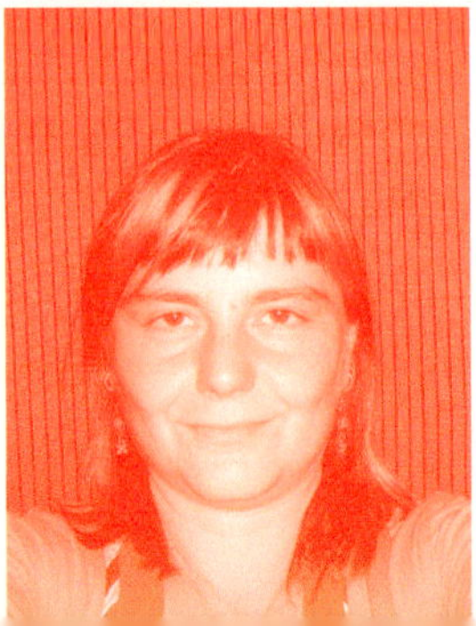
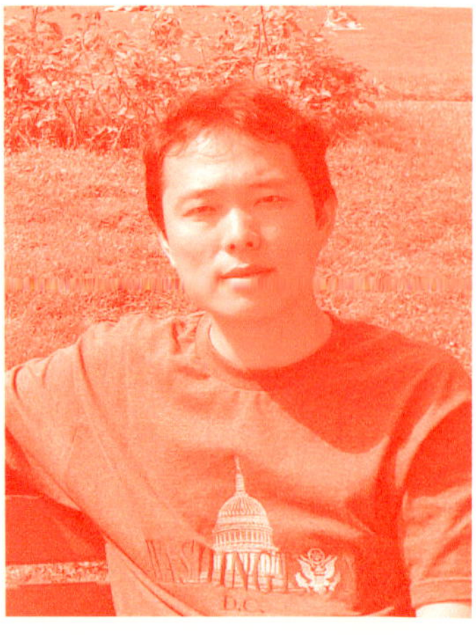

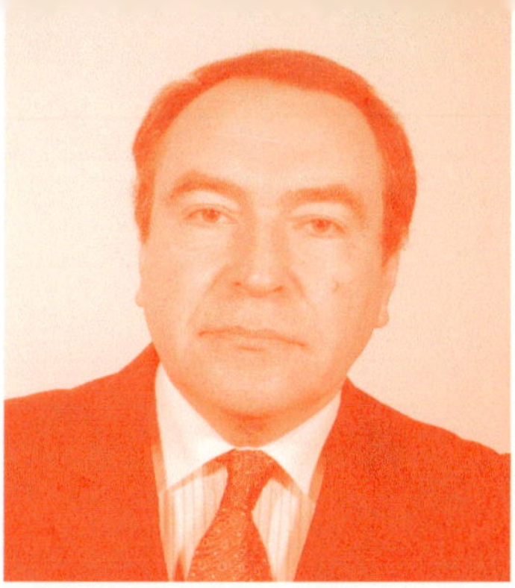
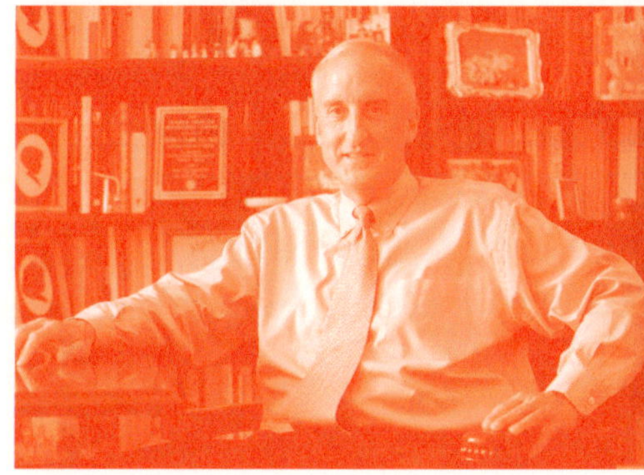
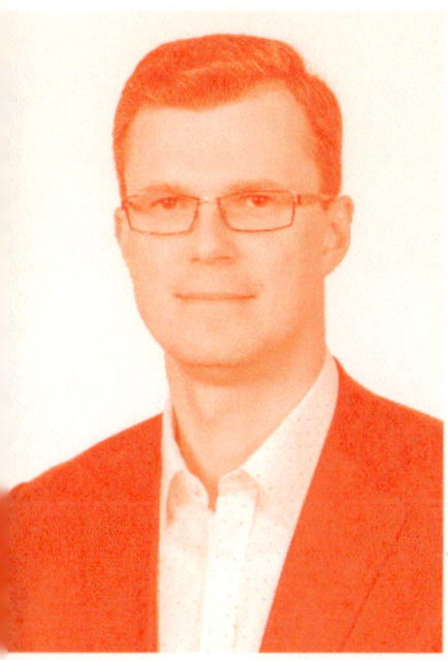
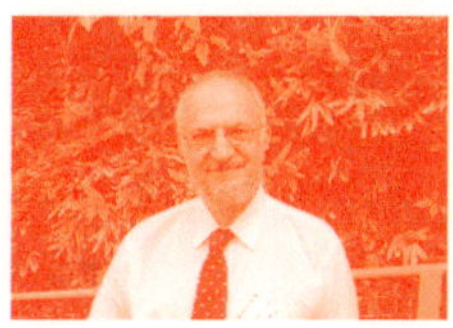
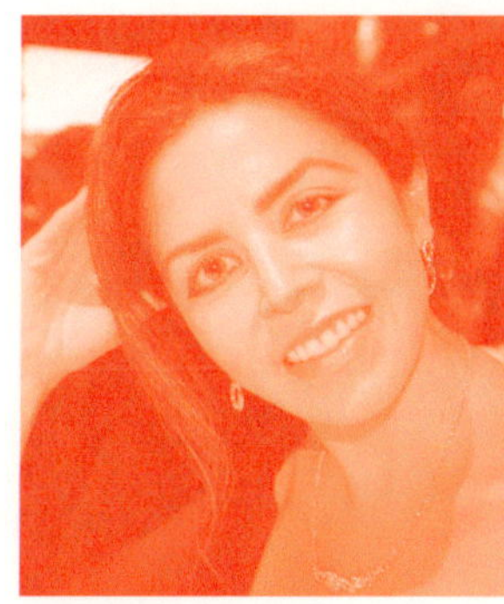

Supporting open minds since 2005

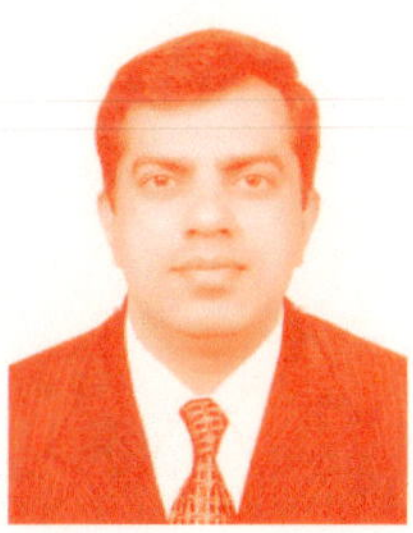
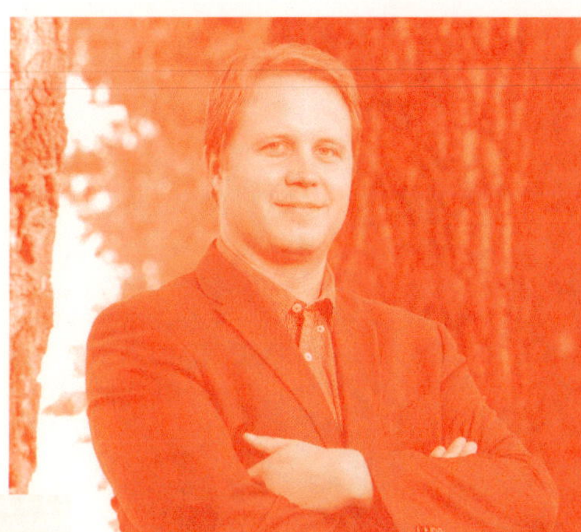
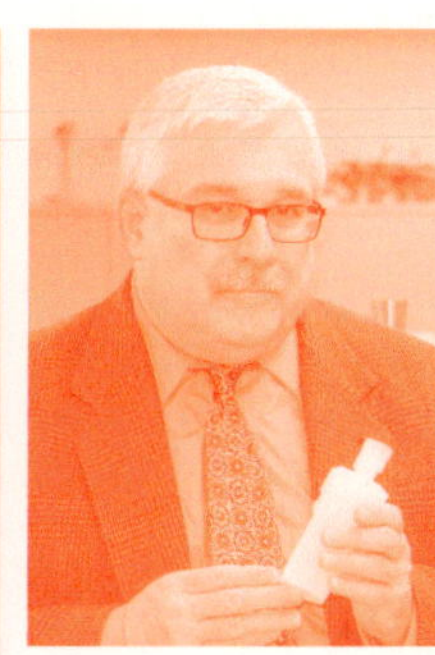
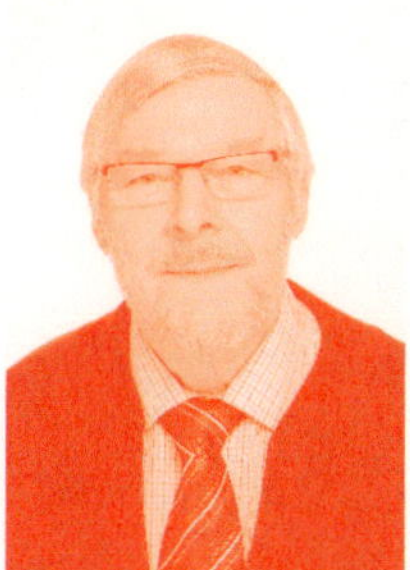
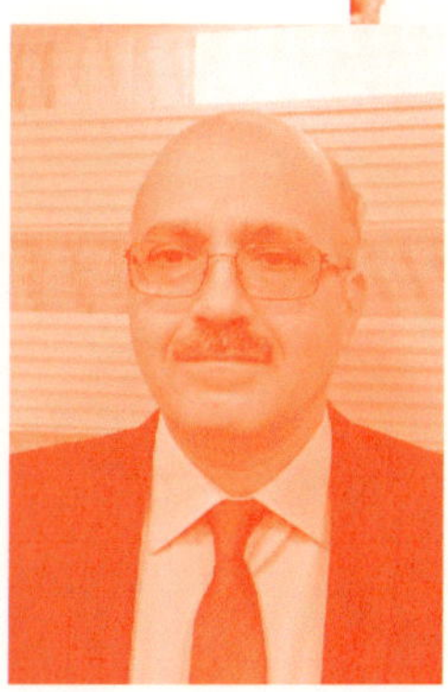
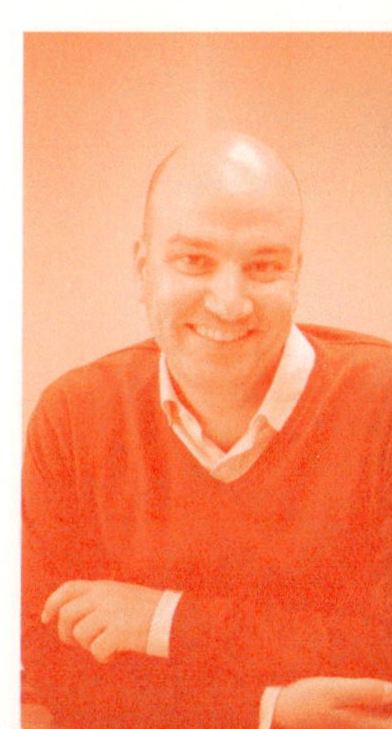
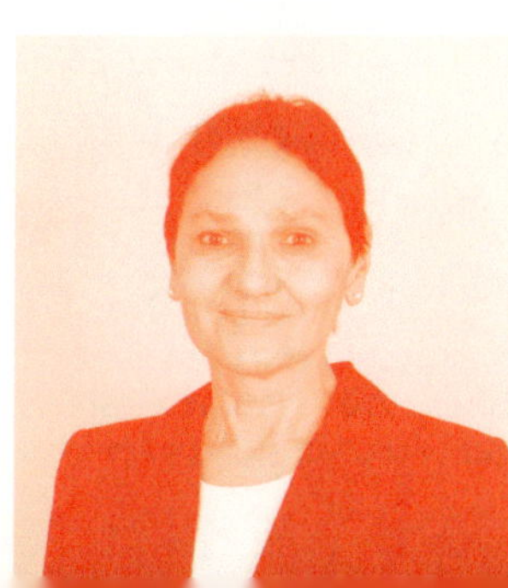

Data Acquisition - Recent Advances and Applications in Biomedical Engineering
http://dx.doi.org/10.5772/intechopen.87796
Edited by Bartłomiej Płaczek

Part of IntechOpen Book Series: Biomedical Engineering, Volume 9
Book Series Editor: Robert Koprowski

Contributors
Namik Tahir Abdullayev, Khadija Ramiz Ahmadova, Ali Usama Syed, Neelum Yousaf Sattar, Zareena Kausar, Ulrich H.P. Fischer-Hirchert, Sabrina Hoppstock, Peter Kußmann, Isabell Steuding, Gulcicek Dere, David Cheneler, Lucy Spain, Bartłomiej Płaczek

First published in London, United Kingdom, 2021 by IntechOpen
IntechOpen is the global imprint of INTECHOPEN LIMITED, registered in England and Wales, registration number: 11086078, 5 Princes Gate Court, London, SW7 2QJ, United Kingdom
Printed in Croatia

British Library Cataloguing-in-Publication Data
A catalogue record for this book is available from the British Library

Additional hard and PDF copies can be obtained from orders@intechopen.com

Data Acquisition - Recent Advances and Applications in Biomedical Engineering
Edited by Bartłomiej Płaczek
p. cm.
Print ISBN 978-1-83968-036-6
Online ISBN 978-1-83968-037-3
eBook (PDF) ISBN 978-1-83968-038-0
ISSN 2631-5343

For EU product safety concerns:
IN TECH d.o.o., Prolaz Marije Krucifikse Kozulić 3, 51000 Rijeka, Croatia, info@intechopen.com or visit our website at intechopen.com.

IntechOpen Book Series
Biomedical Engineering
Volume 9

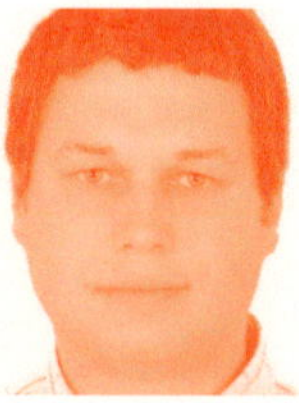

Bartłomiej Płaczek, MSc (2002), Ph.D. (2005), Habilitation (2016), is a professor at the University of Silesia, Institute of Computer Science, Poland, and an expert from the National Centre for Research and Development. His research interests include sensor networks, smart sensors, intelligent systems, and image processing with applications in healthcare and medicine. He is the author or co-author of more than seventy papers in peer-reviewed journals and conferences as well as the co-author of several books. He serves as a reviewer for many scientific journals, international conferences, and research foundations. Since 2010, Dr. Placzek has been a reviewer of grants and projects (including EU projects) in the field of information technologies.

Editor of Volume 9:
Bartłomiej Płaczek
Institute of Computer Science, University of Silesia
Sosnowiec, Poland

Book Series Editor:
Robert Koprowski
University of Silesia, Poland

Scope of the Series

Biomedical engineering is one of the fastest growing interdisciplinary branches of science and industry. The combination of electronics and computer science with biology and medicine has resulted in improved patient diagnosis, reduced rehabilitation time and better quality of life. Nowadays, all medical imaging devices, medical instruments or new laboratory techniques are the result of the cooperation of specialists in various fields. The series of biomedical engineering books covers such areas of knowledge as chemistry, physics, electronics, medicine and biology. This series is intended for doctors, engineers and scientists involved in biomedical engineering or those wanting to start working in this field.

Contents

Preface

Data acquisition is a process of sampling real-world phenomena to collect data that can be manipulated by a computer and software. Data acquisition systems include sensors that convert physical parameters to an electrical signal and utilize computer network technologies for data transfers. Recent advances in biomedical data acquisition systems have led to innovative applications in medical diagnosis, healthcare, and assisted living. The emerging solutions enable the non-invasive and continuous acquisition of valuable biomedical data. Moreover, the collected data can be exchanged using networked systems and analyzed in real time at remote locations.

This book provides insight into the recent advances and applications of biomedical data acquisition technology. It consists of six chapters, each focusing on a specific innovative application.

Chapter 1 concisely reviews several solutions that utilize network-connected sensors for patient activity recognition and monitoring of physiological parameters in healthcare. The considered technological solutions include smart sensors, wireless body sensor networks, and visual sensor networks. The chapter discusses the operation of these networked systems to demonstrate their advantages from the perspective of biomedical data acquisition for representative application examples.

Chapter 2 is devoted to ambient assisted-living systems that can support people in their daily routines by using different types of sensors, mobile devices, computers, communication networks, and software applications. The authors present a data analysis framework that monitors complex patient situations in real time using a web application and a set of sensors. The implemented sensors measure heart rate and breathing rate, analyze gait, and determine the temperature, humidity, and volatile organic compounds of air in the room. Moreover, the proposed system controls an active prosthetic foot to adapt it to the floor covering automatically. The chapter demonstrates that the components of the ambient assisted-living system can communicate with low latency via a heterogeneous network that integrates WiFi, Bluetooth, Gigabit LAN, and 4G+ communication.

Chapter 3 considers acoustic sensor applications for monitoring the joints of the human body. The authors review the use of acoustic emission measurements and vibroarthrography in osteoarthritis diagnosis. These methods' main advantages include the possibility of non-invasive and radiation-free monitoring of variations in joint structure and evaluation of osteoarthritis progression. It is suggested that the acoustic approach could be competitive to state-of-the-art radiographic and magnetic resonance imaging techniques.

Chapter 4 presents a method for controlling advanced prosthetic devices, with the use of an aneural–machine interface. In this method, the introduced data acquisition system translates the human brain's neural activity into control commands for prostheses. Specifically, functional near-infrared spectroscopy was used to acquire data that enable the generation of the control commands for a three degrees-of-freedom prosthetic arm. The experimental results show that popular classification algorithms (artificial neural network and linear discriminant analysis) can be used to predict various arm motions based on the functional near-infrared spectroscopy signals. It is demonstrated that this approach enables the design of improved prostheses for amputees.

Chapter 5 proposes a method to extract informative parameters from the electrocardiogram signal for diagnosing the state of the cardiovascular system. The authors use flicker-noise spectroscopy to analyze correlation relationships in sequences of electrocardiogram irregularities. On this basis, they obtain signal parameters for the normal state of the cardiovascular system and several arrhythmias (ventricular tachycardia, atrial fibrillation, atrial arrhythmia). It is shown that the extracted parameters are useful as input data of an artificial neural network that recognizes pathologies of the cardiovascular system.

Chapter 6 includes an overview of the embedded systems that can be applied for data acquisition in telemedicine, epidemic surveillance, and patient monitoring. The author characterizes popular software and hardware solutions that establish a platform for developing embedded systems. It is also suggested that the embedded systems could contribute to increasing the safety of healthcare workers and patients during the pandemic.

Bartłomiej Płaczek
Institute of Computer Science,
University of Silesia,
Sosnowiec, Poland

Chapter 1

Introductory Chapter: Data Acquisition

Bartłomiej Płaczek

1. Introduction

New biomedical technologies can support faster development of disease treatments, prevention, and diagnostic procedures. They are expected to make significant contributions to the quality of life, improve patient healthcare, and reduce the related costs. Advancement of data acquisition techniques is a key prerequisite for the development in biomedical engineering. Recent advances in data acquisition systems, sensor design, and sensor networks allow collection of large volumes of detailed biomedical data. For instance, body area networks with wireless sensors can be used to non-invasively and continuously monitor several physiological parameters and recognize human activities [1]. Other examples are visual sensor networks for supervision of patients during rehabilitation and Internet of Things (IoT) systems with medical devices connected to the internet that can collect valuable data, enable detailed analysis of symptoms and facilitate remote healthcare. Valuable biomedical data can be also acquired using image processing methods for micrographs analysis [2]. This book intends to provide the reader with an insight into the current state-of-the-art in biomedical data acquisition and focuses on the most important developments in this highly important area.

Few examples of the aforementioned data acquisition techniques are discussed in the introductory chapter. In particular, this chapter concisely reviews the selected approaches that utilize network-connected sensors.

2. Wireless body sensor networks

Different types of sensors can be connected by a wireless body area network (WBAN) in order to monitor various body functions. Usually, the sensors in WBANs are placed on the body. Another approach is to implant small sensors inside the human body. Such approach reduces the impact of WBAN on normal activities of the monitored person. Operations performed by the WBAN sensors include collecting data readings of physical body parameters as well as preprocessing and transmitting the data. The preprocessing operations can be implemented to aggregate, compress or denoise raw sensor readings. A wireless communication is used to transmit the preprocessed data from sensors to a remote destination for further processing or storing. The general concept of WBAN operation is illustrated in **Figure 1**.

The WBAN platforms enable development of ubiquitous medical records in the cloud and on-line healthcare services with disease-alert systems. This technology can contribute to early diagnosis and personalized treatment of patients. It allows the

 IntechOpen

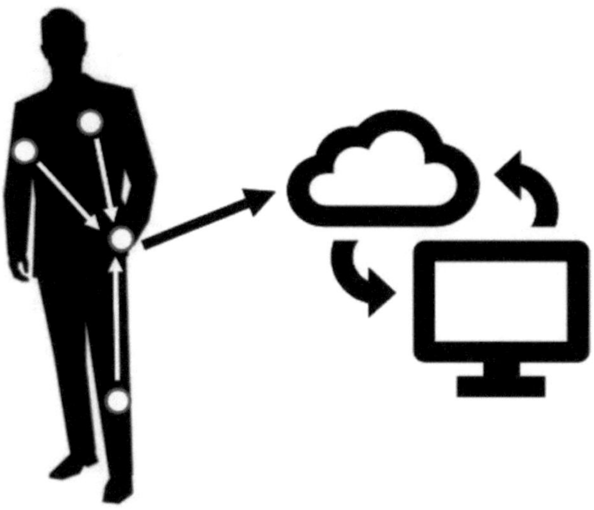

Figure 1.
Wireless body area network (white circles depicts sensors, arrows correspond to data transfers).

patients to be continuously monitored in all locations. In case of health emergency, an alert can be immediately generated to inform the medical staff that urgent intervention is necessary. The data collected by WBANs can also be used to localize person [3] and analyze movement of the body and recognize human activities. On this basis it is possible to develop systems that provide care and security for elderly persons. Moreover, the WBANs found applications in sports for performance monitoring of training activities, rehabilitation, disability assistance, and human–machine interfaces [4].

3. Smart sensors

The above-discussed wireless sensor networks are usually built up with sensors that have the ability to sense physical parameters, perform basic processing tasks and transmit the collected data. More sophisticated solutions are equipped with smart sensors that have extended data processing capabilities. The smart sensors are capable of performing advanced data processing in order to make decisions and recognize relevant events [5]. This kind of sensors may use embedded machine learning algorithms to learn from collected data and to autonomously make assessments or predictions. In case of smart sensors, the data are processed locally. The sensor transmits results of information processing instead of the collected data. This approach leads to reduced data traffic, lower power consumption and latency, as well as to enhanced data privacy.

An example of smart sensor is the solution discussed in [6] which uses a modified support-vector machine classifier for arrhythmia detection based on electrocardiogram signals and for seizure detection based on electroencephalogram signals. It was shown that the above-mentioned detection tasks can be performed by low power wearable sensors in real time.

Another wearable smart sensor was proposed in [7] to detect and categorize cardiac arrhythmias from electrocardiogram readings. A convolutional-recurrent neural network was used in this solution. The neural network was adapted to perform the detection and classification tasks on embedded low-power processors with a small memory footprint.

DOI: http://dx.doi.org/10.5772/intechopen.95019

4. Visual sensor networks

A special type of smart sensors are visual sensors, i.e., camera nodes equipped with embedded processor, and wireless communication module. The smart visual sensors have a number of potential applications, from security and patient monitoring to rehabilitation. For instance, in [8] a visual sensor was introduced for baby behavior monitoring in healthcare centers. This sensor detects abnormal motion of a baby and sends alerts to a user.

Visual sensors can be connected in visual sensor network (VSN). The camera nodes in VSN process image data locally, extract useful information, and exchange the information with other nodes. Using multiple camera nodes in the VSN provides different views of a monitored object, which improves the reliability of the recognized events [9].

In [10] a wireless VSN was proposed for supervision of patient rehabilitation. Results reported in the literature confirms that the VSN concept enables a low cost, light-weight and easy to use monitoring applications that meets tracking and localization needs of rehabilitation centers. An interesting example is the VSN, which was used to collect data for robot automation in rehabilitation of young children [11].

Author details

Bartłomiej Płaczek
Institute of Computer Science, University of Silesia, Sosnowiec, Poland

*Address all correspondence to: placzek.bartlomiej@gmail.com

References

[1] Lewandowski M, Orczyk T, Płaczek B. Human activity detection based on the iBeacon technology. Journal of Medical Informatics & Technologies. 2016:25

[2] Płaczek B, Bułdak RJ, Polaniak R. Automatic immunogold particle detection in transmission electron micrographs of cancer cells. Journal of Medical Imaging and Health Informatics. 2015;**5**(6):1350-1357

[3] Bernas M, Płaczek B. Fully connected neural networks ensemble with signal strength clustering for indoor localization in wireless sensor networks. International Journal of Distributed Sensor Networks. 2015;**11**(12):403242

[4] Meharouech A, Elias J, Mehaoua A. Moving towards body-to-body sensor networks for ubiquitous applications: A survey. Journal of Sensor and Actuator Networks. 2019;**8**(2):27

[5] Lewandowski M, Płaczek B. An Event-Aware Cluster-Head Rotation Algorithm for Extending Lifetime of Wireless Sensor Network with Smart Nodes. Sensors. 2019;**19**(19):4060

[6] Lee KH, Kung SY, Verma N. Low-energy formulations of support vector machine kernel functions for biomedical sensor applications. Journal of Signal Processing Systems. 2012;**69**(3):339-349

[7] Faraone A, Delgado-Gonzalo R. Convolutional-recurrent neural networks on low-power wearable platforms for cardiac arrhythmia detection. In: 2020 2nd IEEE International Conference on Artificial Intelligence Circuits and Systems (AICAS). IEEE; 2020. pp. 153-157

[8] Hussain T, Muhammad K, Khan S, Ullah A, Lee MY, Baik SW. Intelligent baby behavior monitoring using embedded vision in IoT for smart healthcare centers. Journal of Artificial Intelligence and Systems;(15):1, 2019

[9] Soro S, Heinzelman W. A survey of visual sensor networks. Advances in multimedia. 2009

[10] Idoudi M, Bourennane EB, Grayaa K. Wireless visual sensor network platform for indoor localization and tracking of a patient for rehabilitation task. IEEE Sensors Journal. 2018;**18**(14):5915-5928

[11] Kokkoni E, Mavroudi E, Zehfroosh A, Galloway JC, Vidal R, Heinz J, et al. GEARing smart environments for pediatric motor rehabilitation. Journal of NeuroEngineering and Rehabilitation. 2020;**17**(1):16

Chapter 2

Real-Time Capable Sensor Data Analysis-Framework for Intelligent Assistance Systems

Ulrich H.P. Fischer, Sabrina Hoppstock, Peter Kußmann and Isabell Steuding

Abstract

In the industrialized countries, the very old part of the population has been growing rapidly for many years. In the next few years in particular, the age cohort over 65 will increase significantly. This goes hand in hand with illnesses and other physical and cognitive limitations. In order to enable these people to remain in their own homes for as long as possible despite physical and cognitive restrictions, technologies are being used to create ambient assisted living applications. However, most of these systems are neither medically verified nor are latencies short enough, for example, to avoid falls. In order to overcome these problems, a promising approach is to use the new 5G network technology. Combined with a suitable sensor data analysis frame work, the fast care project showed that a real-time situation picture of the patient in the form of an Avatar could be generated. The sensor structure records the heart rate, the breathing rate, analyzes the gait and measures the temperature, the VOC content of the room air, and its humidity. An emergency button has also been integrated. In a laboratory demonstrator, it was shown that the infrastructure realizes a real-time visualization of the sensor data over a heterogeneous network.

Keywords: ambient assisted living technologies, eHealth, eCare, tele-care, real-time networks, vital data acquisition, fast project

1. Introduction

Assistance systems in Ambient Assisted Living and in medical care have to recognize relevant situations, that require fast assistive intervention. Former projects in this field like tecla [1–3] or PAUL [4] have been focused on the application of the new AAL-technologies in AAL test beds to get information about the acceptance level [5, 6] of the technologies and the different new applications for the patients. Additionally, business models [7, 8] have been drafted to realize a successful AAL business area in future.

The clinical established measurement technology for diagnostic, monitoring and risk stratification does not translate directly to the outpatient area (ambulant or domestically environment). The key challenge is, that many relevant situations are only noticeable, when various sensor modalities are merged – such as for discrimination between pathological, emotional [9] or stress induced increase of the heart rate [10]. This is only possible by the use of the combination of multiple different sensors [11]. The same applies to the analysis of joint kinematics of everyday activities, which requires more and inertial sensors with higher accuracy.

The next generation of radio networks (5G) [12] shows the possibility of introducing new possibilities of real-time communication in all areas of life with very low latency and high data rates. One speaks of a so-called tactile Internet. People come into contact with their surroundings through their senses, which involve several different reaction times. Here, muscular, audio-visual and tactile response times are of particular importance. The typical muscular response time is around 1 second, that of the hearing at 100 ms, while the visual response time is in the range of 10 ms [13].

In the case of active control of an object, such as a car or a machine, the information must first be recorded while a reaction must be carried out at the same time. The well-known use of a touch screen requires that you move your finger in a controlled manner across the screen. It is therefore necessary that the touch screen can achieve a response time of less than 1 ms in order not to produce any noticeable delay in the visual impression. In the case of an active prothesis, which was applied in this study, the response time must be below 10 ms to achieve a practical application basis for its use in daily life. Therefore, fast sensor data-frameworks are needed to analyze the conditions of real-time identification and subsequently provide a medical valid corresponding assistance [12, 14].

The aim of the fast care project was to develop a real-time sensor data analysis framework [9] for intelligent assistance systems in the area of Ambient Assisted Living (AAL), eHealth, mHealth, tele-rehabilitation and tele-care. It provides a medically valid, integrated real-time situation picture based on a distributed, ad hoc networking, everyday use and energy-efficient sensor infrastructure with a latency of less than several ms. The integrated situation picture that includes physiological, cognitive, kinematic information of the patient is generated by the intelligent fusion of sensor data [15, 16]. It can serve as a basis both for the rapid detection of risks and dangerous situations as well as for everyday use medical assistance systems that autonomously intervene in real time [17, 18] and allows active telemedical feedback [10].

In this chapter of the book, after an introduction, the technical goals and implementation options of a fast sensor network with real-time data analysis are presented followed without contact by the structure of the overall system. In the Section 2, the details of the technological concept such as data fusion and telemetry are presented. All relevant interfaces for real-time applications are discussed in detail. In the following section, the hardware, sensors/actuators and the specific installation of the demonstrator in laboratory operation are discussed. In the following part, details of the individual sensor systems and the corresponding visualization of the sensor data presented by an Avatar are distinguished. In the Section 3, the acceptance test for the use of the sensor components of the demonstration are analyzed and discussed. Finally, a summary with a view of upcoming developments will be given at the end.

2. Technical goals and solutions

2.1 System setup

The basis of a medical valid - integrated real-time picture of the situation is an ad hoc interconnected sensor infrastructure. Its latency period should be very fast to fulfill the boundaries of a haptive working network. Here, physiological, cognitive and kinematic information of a patient are captured with the help of intelligent sensor data fusion. These data can be combined to provide an integrated picture of the patient's physical and mental situation. In this way, it should be ensured that the framework can be used for applications, in which feedback has to be embedded synchronically. This can be realized in visual, auditive, tactile or proprioceptive string of perception, such as in the field of support of motor function and kinematics for the rehabilitation and for active prosthetics and orthotics.

Figure 1 shows an overview of the system concept of the project approach for an integrated sensor infrastructure in the home of an elderly person. It consists of GPS data, air pressure and temperature data, vital parameters, cameras, optical sensors and so-called inertial sensors (IMU) together.

These sensor data are summarized in real-time and buffered in a database system. From this database, an integrated real-time situation analysis is generated that touches on three areas of human life: firstly, the kinematic data such as localization, movement and posture. The second area is the cognitive sub-area with awareness, emotionality and mental clarity. The third subsection deals with the physiological data in which cardiovascular metabolic and neurological data can be recorded and analyzed.

This entirety of the data in the home of the living person can be evaluated integratively and can accordingly provide a precise analysis of his health. In this project, apart from the emotional and neurological aspects, all the addressed areas were recorded and evaluated. After evaluating the situation analysis, actuators are implemented for rehabilitation, in a special case of an active prosthesis of the foot, which can adjust different heel heights, automatic adaptation to different floor conditions or rapid walking. Furthermore, the client should be provided with a real-time display of his vital parameters as a so-called Smart Home Assistant, which can give a helpful health support to the client.

For a real-time application, it is necessary that the latency times between sensor detection and actuator actuation are less than several Milliseconds. This ensures a so-called haptic functionality of the system and can be achieved with the help of new radio technologies and fast network technologies such as FTTH and the fifth

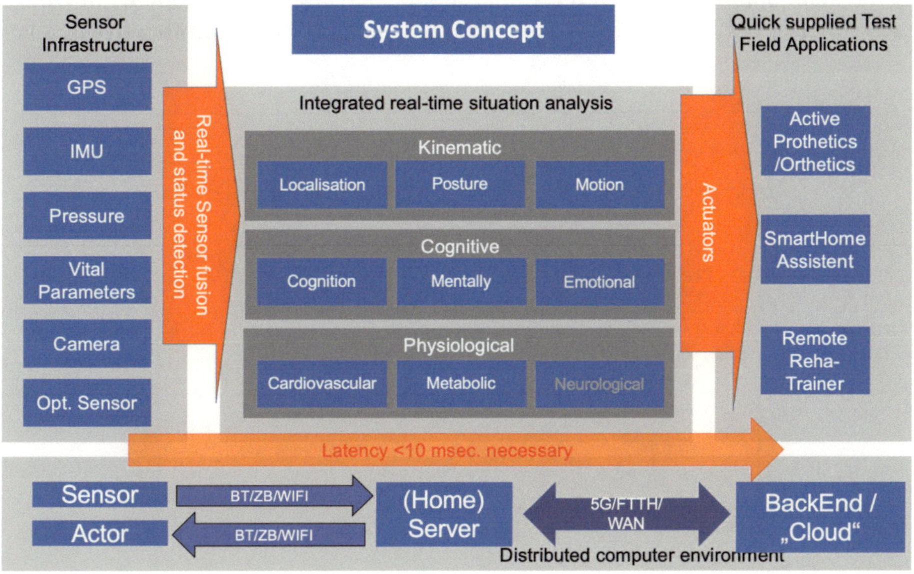

Figure 1.
Integrated system concept.

generation of mobile radio networks (5G). To ensure private data security, all data is stored and evaluated in a so-called home server which is situated in the client's apartment. Further intervention options are possible by a secure cloud connection to medical services or the system administrators for possible updates of the sensor and actuator components.

The challenge of a distributed, real-time medical sensor technology and signal processing is to be processed by means of sensor-based data processing and sensor hubs, optical sensors, hardware system optimization, the development of distributed systems as well as by interface network sensors. The focus of the project was on the intelligent fusion of sensor and actuator data as well as the evaluation and delivery in real-time. In order to meet this objective, the following developments took place in the Ambient Assisted Living (AAL)-Lab of the Harz University of Applied Sciences in Wernigerode (**Figure 2**).

- Analysis of requirements
- Data acquisition
- Data analysis
- Data fusion
- Acceptance analysis
- Situation detection and assistance in real-time

The objective of a distributed, real-time medical sensor technology and signal processing is to get an evaluation of the patient's situation from the available data in real-time. The main application focuses in the area of the application of orthopedic devices. For example, the optimization process of the leg prosthesis` damping members and active foot positioning points shall be executed online. Currently, these parameters are performed offline and hand-made by orthopedic technicians with variable quality. This often leads to suboptimal adapted orthopedic devices; whose functionality and efficacy are correspondingly limited and therefore to an

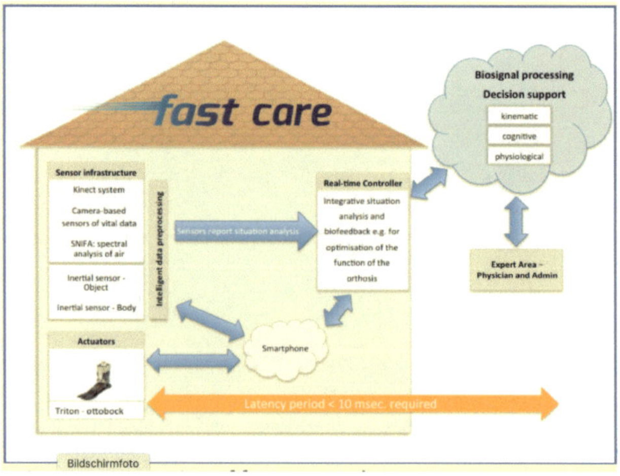

Figure 2.
Application of fast care real-time sensor system.

unsatisfactory rehabilitation outcome. This system approach of the sensor integration into an active foot prothesis is called a real-time active prosthetics/orthotics - time controller. Another project section describes the online execution of the estimation of cognitive condition, the motion analysis for rehabilitation and cardiopulmonary performance.

2.2 Technological concept

Based on the project goals, the technical and content requirements of the technological topics to be worked on were specified, categorized and summarized by the individual partners. The basic requirements are listed in the following areas:

1. Hardware/sensors,

2. Network,

3. Data analysis,

4. Actuators/intervention/feedback

The system diagram of the research approach of the fast care framework is shown in the **Figure 3**. The fast care framework is the technical basis for the realization of the fast care project, which implements the fusion of heterogeneous sensors via heterogeneous networks. The basic idea of the fast care framework is to derive a condition from the past and the current states of the sensory data using different newly developed sensor applications, including the following areas and interfaces (see **Figure 3**). From the network topological representation, a breakdown of the used network interfaces was made, specified by the project partners. Based on this, a suitable communication protocol was selected regarding the individual implementations. Communication via MQTT forms the basis of the used communication between the sensor-applications and the real-time controller depicted in **Figure 3**. In the left side of the figure, the sensor-applications are situated, consisting of a Kinect system for motion data, inertial motion units (IMU) for the detection of movements of body and objects in a fixed sequence for the analysis of a workout in a kitchen, motion sensors/actuators in an active intelligent prothesis, a camera based heart rate and breathe sensor, and finally a special sensor of volatile organic components in the room air. Prothesis, body and objects sensors are connected via smartphone and Bluetooth low energy. While the smartphone transfers the data to the real-time controller.

In total, the seven sensor components are listed there on the left. The active prosthesis, the heart rate measurement, the respiratory rate measurement, the detection of VOC components in the breathing air, the detection of movement in the room and the measurement of room temperature and humidity, as well as the use of the emergency button, uses the corresponding network structure according to the blocks shown in the sketch.

After the individual implementations of the interfaces a suitable software communication server was selected. The MQTT protocol [19] was implemented using a real-time capable Linux variant. Suitable hardware was procured by the project partner of the Harz University of Applied Sciences, a suitable operating system was installed and the MQTT software server "mosquitto" [20] was installed and configured. The definition of topics (message channels) and the specification of the data formats were necessary for smooth communication of the individual partner realizations "in-itself" and "with each other." A detailed description of the

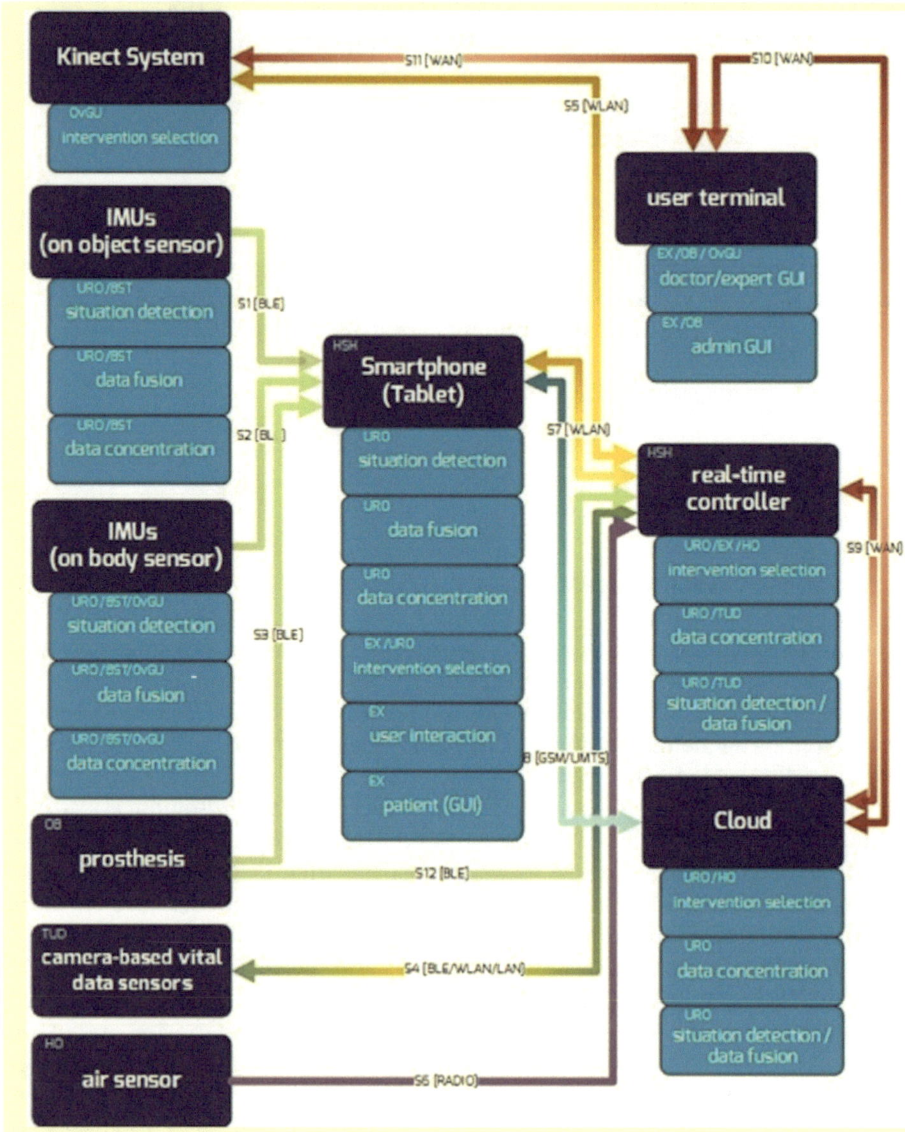

Figure 3.
Network topology.

communication formats between the sensors built by the partners and the MQTT server can be found in the final design plan of the fast care project [21].

At the beginning of the project, the communication protocols that should be used between the individual project partners for data exchange have been discussed and clearly defined (see **Table 1**). The interfaces for the network used in the project are essentially the Bluetooth LE transmission, the Wi-Fi transmission and the wired transmission via Ethernet 802.3. Furthermore, wireless transmission via LTE or 4G plus was used by several partners. This resulted in a very broad transmission application scenario. An overview of the transmission technology of the sensor infrastructure to the real-time controller and the forwarding to the real-time visualization is depicted in **Figure 4**.

N.	Description	Partner		Technology	
S1	Communication interface between IMU's (Object) and a smartphone	URO BST	HSH	IMU (Object) Bluetooth SMART	Smartphone Bluetooth SMART READY
S2	Communication interface between IMUs (body) and a smartphone	URO BST OvGu	HSH	IMU (Body) Bluetooth SMART	Smartphone Bluetooth SMART READY
S3	Communication interface between a prosthesis and a smartphone	OBO	HSH	Prothesis Bluetooth SMART	Smartphone Bluetooth SMART READY
S4	Communication interface between the camera-based vital sensors and the real-time controller	TUD	HSH	Camera based Vital parameter sensors Bluetooth SMART, WiFi, IEEE	Real-time controller Bluetooth SMART READY, WiFi, IEEE
S5	Communication interface between the Kinect system and the real-time controller	OvGU	HSH	Kinect-System WiFi	Real-time controller WiFi
S6	Communication interface between the VCO air sensor and the real-time controller	HO	HSH	VOC air sensor WiFi	Real-time controller WiFi
S7	Communication interface between the smartphone and the real-time controller	HSH	HSH	Smartphone WiFi	Real-time controller WiFi
S8	Communication system between the smartphone and the cloud system	HSH	EXE HO	Communication system 4G +	Cloud-System 4G +
S9	Communication system between the real-time controller and the cloud system	HSH	URO HO	Real-time controller WAN IEEE	Cloud-System WAN IEEE
S10	Communication system between the cloud system and the end device	URO HO	EXE OBO OvGu	Cloud-System WAN IEEE	Terminal WAN IEEE
S11	Communication system between the Kinect system and the end device	OvGu	OvGu	Kinect-System WAN IEEE	Terminal WAN IEEE
S12	Communication system between the prosthesis and the real-time controller	OBO	HSH/ OBO	Prothesis Bluetooth SMART	Real-time controller Bluetooth SMART READY

Table 1.
Overview of network interface parts used in fast care.

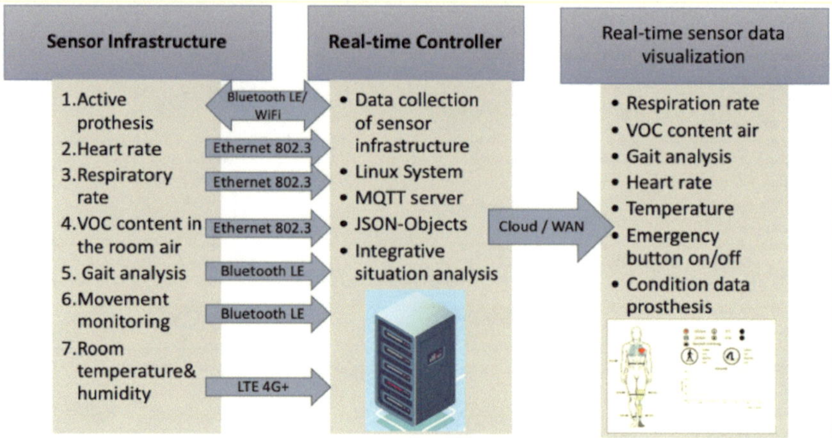

Figure 4.
Network infrastructure [22].

After the data has been transferred to the real-time controller, the data is available in the form of JSON objects that were stored on the Linux system of the server. At the same time, an integrative situation analysis of the sensor data is carried out and the corresponding information is transferred to the real-time visualization via the public network to a cloud server, which generates a website with the correspondingly evaluated real-time data in the form of an Avatar.

2.3 Hardware, sensors, actors

In this part all of the hardware components which have been developed in the project are described. On the one hand, this includes sensors with the task of capturing a physical measured variable like motion, VOC gas, heart rate, etc. Furthermore, sensor modules have been developed with implemented combined sensors which form a functional unit with actuators e.g. the electronically controllable lower leg prosthesis. For a better overview of the components used by the individual partners, a matrix of the use of all partners and their network interfaces was created. (See **Table 2**).

	Kinect	IMUs (Body)	IMUs (Object)	Prothesis	Camera	VOC Sen.	Smart phone	Real-time controller	Cloud	Terminal
HSH							+	+	+	
TUD					+			++	+	
OvGU	+	+								+
URO		+	+				++++	+++	+++	
EX							+++	+	+	++
BST		+	+							
OBO				+						++
HO						+		+	+	

Table 2.
Types of hardware components used by the cooperation partners.

In the following subsections all of the used hardware and all sensors/actors are collected and described.

2.3.1 AAL lab installation

Rapid and intelligent sensors and actuators, an improvement of motion pattern recognition and intelligent algorithms for real-time network integration in three demonstrators of the AAL-Lab serve as solution approaches. Within the fast care project, a real-time network integration with demonstrators is to be carried out at the AAL-Lab of the Harz University. The various partial results of the project partners have been collected and integrated in the AAL-Lab. The integration at the AAL-Lab will be performed with the focus on user friendliness and the interaction with him by means of a show flat. **Figure 5** illustrates the realized structure of the AAL-Lab with various elements for monitoring and evaluation of the measured vital data. The lab includes the following parts: Sensors on the walls: Pulse, Blood pressure, breathing frequency, Motion/position, VOC breath analysis, e-rehabilitation workout and the real-time controller PC.

In **Figure 6** you can see the laboratory, including a sofa, several armchairs, a bed and all the sensor components that were attached to the room, as shown in the **Figure 5**. The room has been deliberately designed like an old room to create a pleasant atmosphere for the examinations. After the technology was installed, the acceptance tests were carried out in this environment.

2.3.2 E-rehabilitation system

The Kinect sensor used by the Otto von Guericke University in fast care is a physical device with depth sensor technology, integrated color camera, infrared transmitter and microphone array that detects the position and movement of people and voices. **Table 2** shows the data of the KINECT depth sensor, while **Figure 7** shows the workout scene. The application is to make a therapeutically workout with the patient and give him in real-time information and helpful feedback to move him

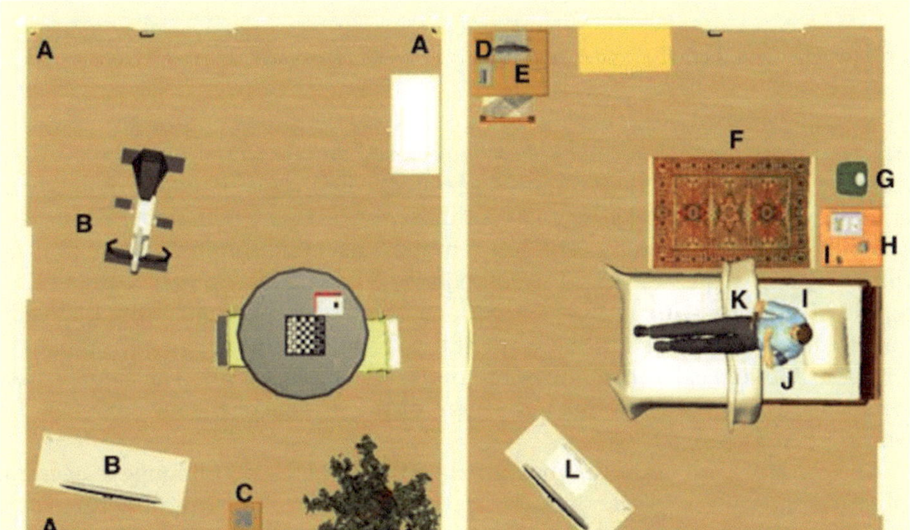

Figure 5.
AAL lab of the Harz university; sketch of installations; (a) sensors on the walls: Pulse, blood pressure, breathing frequency, skin resistance, motion/position, VOC breath analysis, (b) E-rehabilitation, (c) real-time controller.

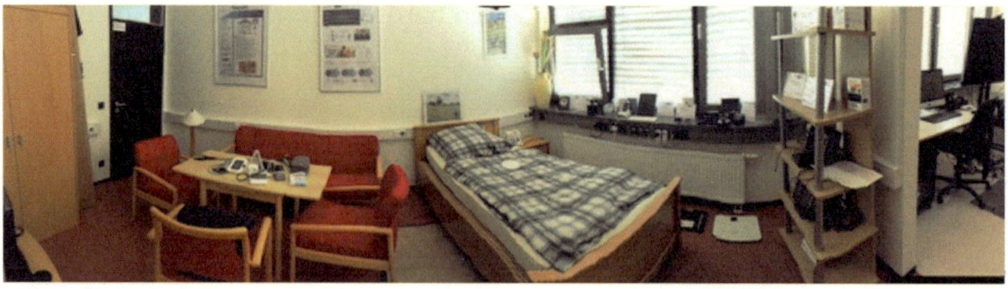

Figure 6.
Photograph of AAL lab.

in the right way. Additionally, a gait analysis [23, 24] can be performed by the use of IMUs positioned at the feet, shown in **Figure 7**. More detailed information can be found by Stoutz et al. in [25] (**Table 3**).

2.3.3 Inertial measurement unit (IMU)

The IMU used by the project partners "Otto Bock HealthCare GmbH", "Otto von Guericke University" and "University of Rostock" describes an initial measuring unit. It is a self-contained measuring system that continuously records, analyzes, and, if necessary, pre-processes defined physical parameters (e.g. movement, acceleration, pressure, etc.) and forwards them to downstream communication and network protocols (see **Figure 8**). A distinction is made between two application modes. On the one hand, the IMUs on an object e.g. be installed in a kitchen appliance [26], which describes the use of "IMU on object" and provides measurement data for further analysis. Another area of application is the use of an IMU through suitable holders on the body of a person, which in turn describes the use of the "initial sensor on body" and also provides measurement data for further analysis [27, 28]. The project partner "Bosch Sensortec GmbH" [29, 30] developed and produces the IMU's used in the fast care project [31].

2.3.4 Camera-based vital parameter sensor

The camera-based vital sensors [32, 33] used by the project partner of the "Technical University Dresden" [34–36] are based on one or more camera systems with an associated, spectrally controllable lighting system and generate a spatial image of the surroundings as a database for further evaluations. Camera-based photoplethysmography (cbPPG) remotely detects the volume pulse of cardiac ejection in the peripheral circulation. The system does measure the heart rate, the breath rate with a camera system contactless in real time. More detailed information's are described in the work of the Technical University of Dresden, Institute of Biomedical Technologies of Zaunseder et al. [37, 38]. The camera-based system records the change in the movement of the surface of the face in a fast data recording (see **Figure 9**).

The exposure with an LED light source with a special spectral range is necessary to obtain a particularly good contrast. The raw image data are sent directly to a controller and evaluated there. The evaluated data (heart rate, respiratory rate) are transferred directly as a JSON object to the real-time controller via Ethernet cabling at 1 Gb/s and stored there in the MQTT server. The representation of the respiratory rate and the heart rate is then realized in real time in the Avatar (see Sensor Data Visualization 2.4).

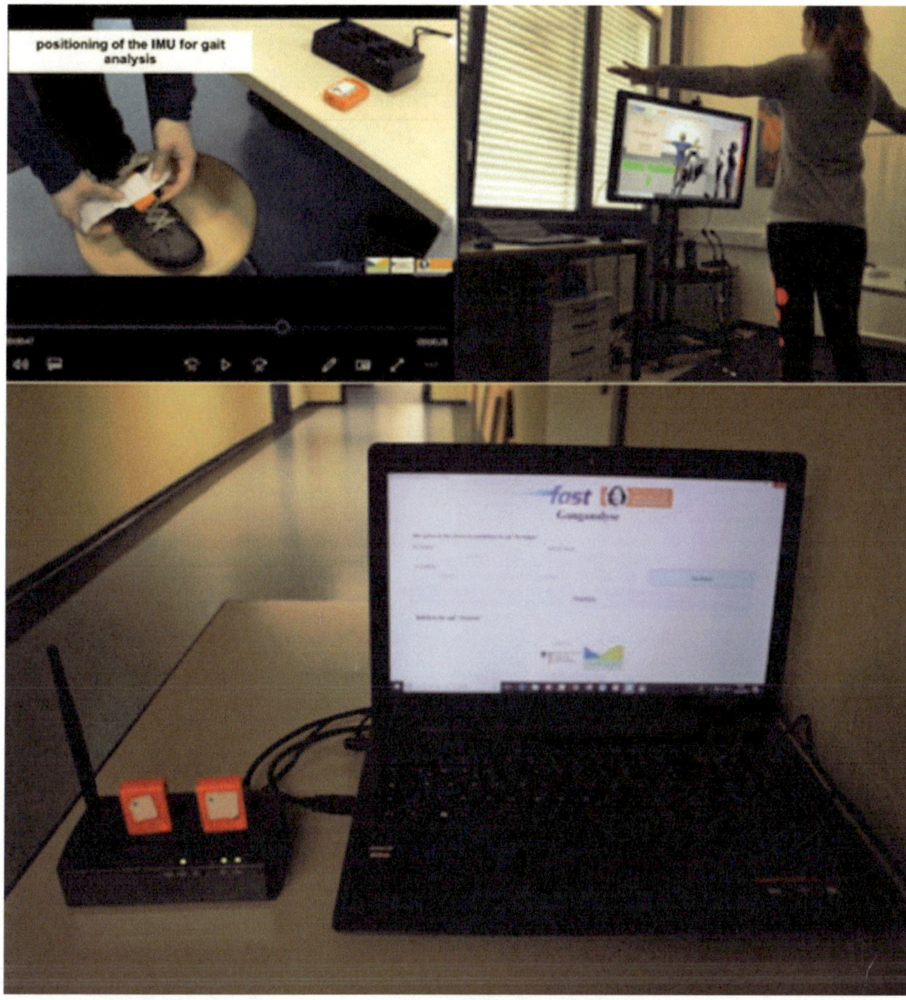

Figure 7.
Setup of the gait measurements for e-rehabilitation of Otto von Guericke university; above left: IMU application at the feet; above right: Therapeutic movements with avatar; lower middle: Presentation of gait analysis measurement.

Feature	Description	
Depth sensor 512 × 424, 30 Hz FOV: 70 × 60 One-Modus: 0.5–4.5 m	Optimized 3D visualization, detection of smaller objects in particular and stable body tracking	
1080p-Color Camera 30 Hz (15 Hz in poor lighting conditions)	Camera with 1080p resolution	
Neue aktive Infrarot-Funktionen 512 × 424, 30 Hz	IR functions for lighting independent observations	
Multi-Array-Microphone	Four microphones etc. to find the sound source and the direction of the audio wave	
Interfaces	Kinect	AUX (USB)
	Kinect2	AUX (USB)

Table 3.
Data of the used KINECT sensor system for e-rehabilitation.

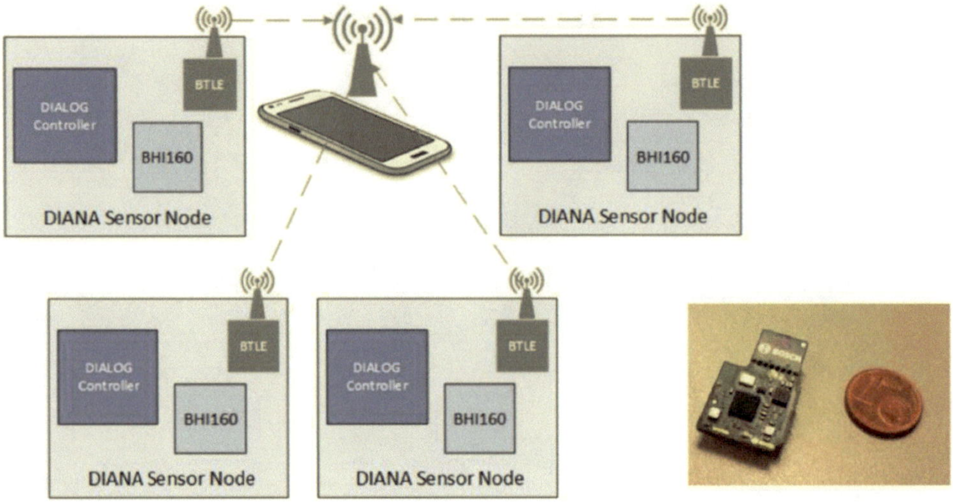

Figure 8.
Structure of the inertial measurement unit network.

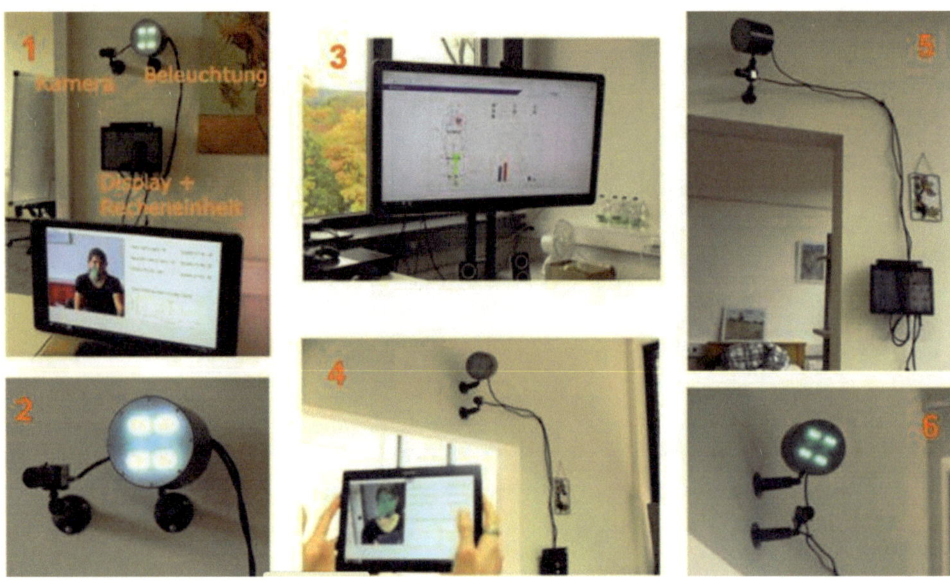

Figure 9.
Camera-based vital sensors, 1 measurement unit, 2: Camera and lighting system 1, 3: Central display of real-time measurement 4: Measurement system 1 while application, 5: Measurement system 2 in while application, 6: Camera and lighting system 2.

2.3.5 VOC air sensor

As part of the BMBF-funded "fast care" project, HarzOptics GmbH [39] has developed components for a distributed sensor network for the spectroscopic analysis of air. The sensor system analyzes the air in a room by measuring the optical spectral content of volatile organic components (VOC) [39–42]. Special absorptions of VOC gases are analyzed, which indicate the beginning of clinical pictures. In addition to assessing the quality of indoor air for AAL applications, this system is also to be used for the detection of VOC in breathing gas. Since the presence of certain VOCs in exhaled air enables conclusions to be drawn about

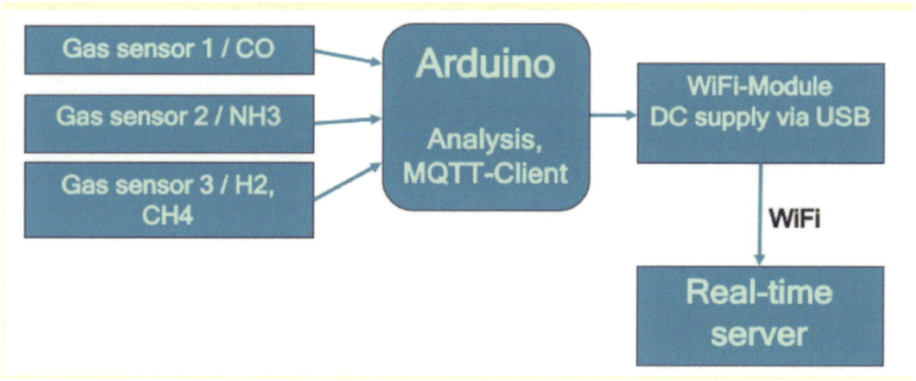

Figure 10.
VOC sensor setup.

diseases such as lung cancer or metabolic disorders, the integration of a non-invasive permanent gas analysis in real-time medical care is becoming possible, also in view of increasing bandwidths and decreasing latency times [39].

The air sensor is part of a more complex system, the basic mode of operation of which can be seen in **Figure 10**. Data recorded by a sensor (e.g. CO2 concentration) are transferred as (voltage) values to an Arduino board, which converts the values into volume concentrations, converts the data generated from it into an MQTT-compliant format and transmits it to a real-time server. The data is displayed using a special real time Avatar sketch which is presented in chapter 4.10 in more detail. If limits are exceeded, a warning or recommendation is issued (e.g. "Please open window and ventilate" or "Please consult a doctor"). In addition to the data from this sensor, the MQTT server also receives data from other sensors that have been developed by other project partners. These are also visualized in the Avatar figure.

After the spectrum could not be recorded using an optical spectrometer due to a lack of sensitivity, an alternative setup with laser sources was implemented. The wavelengths used here correspond to the previously determined absorptions of the relevant substances and are recorded by a broadband optical sensor. If the substances sought are present in the air, the light from the laser source is attenuated in accordance with the concentration, which reduces the voltage values at the sensor output and the volume concentration can be determined. The temperature sensitivity of the sensor and amplifier is still causing problems.

2.3.6 Active prothesis

Under the catchphrase "active prosthesis", "Otto Bock HealthCare GmbH" summarizes its IMUs worn on the body, an associated analysis and evaluation unit and the control of an active prosthetic foot. The aim is to map an automatic adjustment of an active prosthetic foot using a long-term measurement of a gait analysis based on the foot, knee and joint angle. The realization of the complete measurement system is described in more details by Albrecht-Laatsch in [43]. The current status quo for the adaptation of prostheses is that clients rarely come to adapt their prostheses for rehabilitation and check-ups. Therefore, the prosthesis is usually only adapted for one type of gait. In addition, developers rarely speak to users, so that little everyday problems flow into development.

The goal of the development the active prothesis in the fast care project was to get a better picture of the real prosthesis usage, as well as to make it easier and faster to adapt to the real needs of the user. This was achieved with a remote connection of the active prosthetic foot used for remote diagnosis and automatic adaptation to the conditions of use.

Implementation was achieved with the help of motion sensors (IMU), the measured values of which were used both locally and remotely. This eliminates the need for a regular visit to the gait laboratory and the long-term recording takes place in a relaxed environment. In addition, incorrect movement patterns can be recognized and corrected early. The adaptation takes place automatically and can be initiated from a "remote" location. With the active prosthetic foot, the heel height and the active aisle support could be automatically adjusted by the software. This reduces fatigue, as the engine pushes the legs off. The support is regulated depending on the speed. For experts in the laboratory, the gait diagram is displayed remotely in real time, and further parameters of the prosthesis can be remotely adjusted by the experts in fine tuning mode. The test of the automatic adaptation of the was performed in the laboratory which is depicted in the working scene of **Figure 11**.

2.3.7 Bluetooth beacons

The University of Rostock uses "bulky BLE Beacons" to locate its IMUs in the room [27, 28]. These beacons are distributed in a fixed position in the room and allow the IMU's to make statements about movements in the space of people and their acceleration via a field strength measurement. The sensors provide information about using a kitchen task assessment dataset. This dataset contains normal behavior as well as erroneous behavior due to dementia, recorded with wearable sensors as well as with sensors attached to objects. The scene of the application of the kitchen task workout is depicted **Figure 12**.

In this workout, a test client prepares a pudding meal that is clearly defined in a few simple steps. The process goes through the compilation of the ingredients, the cooking itself to completion and decanting the pudding into several cups. All subprocesses are analyzed in detail and provided with appropriate help if the wrong ingredients are used or the wrong wooden spoon, while all objects in the environment which the person is working, are connected with IMU sensors.

The kitchen task is created by a semantic annotation scheme. This scheme gives information about the observed motions and the errors while performing the workout. The data format splits in sensor and video data. The video data are collected by several cameras while the sensor data are collecting parallel to the video several accelerations from the IMU sensors fixed at the body worn sensors and

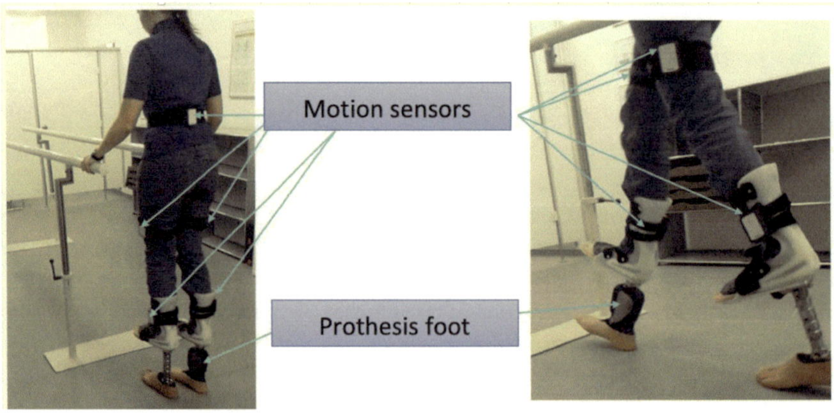

Figure 11.
Active prothesis motion sensor with feedback for gait optimization.

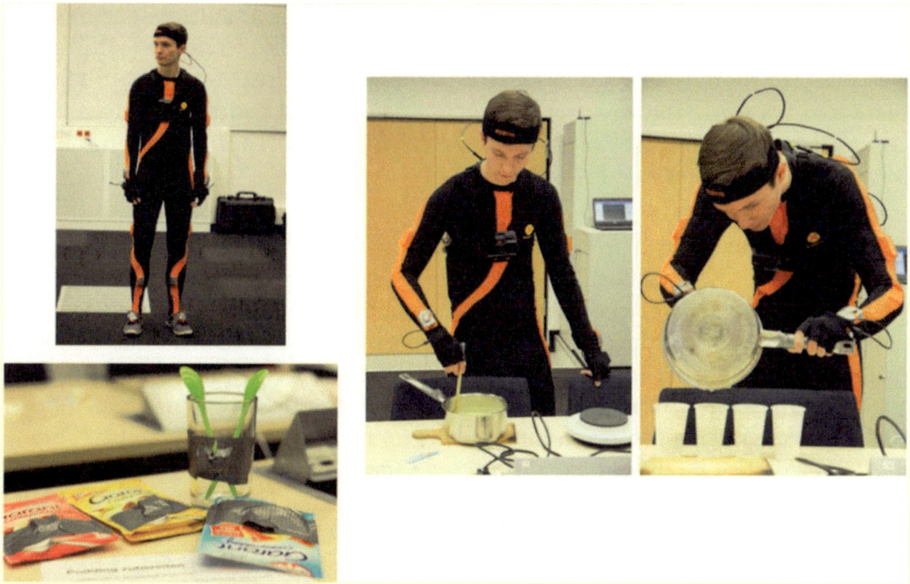

Figure 12.
Motion analysis of a cooking process with IMUs with inference method at university Rostock.

additional from the used objects. The complete data roll consists of several normal and false runs. To get information about the false runs, the clients realized errors in the workout. The data consists of action data as well as the object being manipulated and the client that is working with it. More information about the sensor application to analyze the erroneous behavior from Hein et al. can be found in [44].

2.3.8 Emergency button and temperature/humidity sensors

As an additional sensor system, the Exelonix company implemented an NbIoT sensor as a push button, which transmits its sensor data in JSON format to the real-time server via the public network via the existing 4G + radio network (see **Figure 13**). The emergency is displayed in real time on the visualization server. In the real case, this could then be transmitted to the 24/7 service of a nursing service.

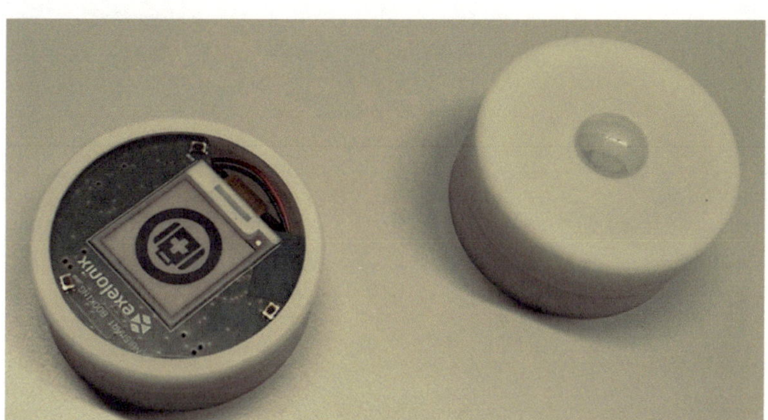

Figure 13.
Sensor modules of Exelonix, left: IoT emergency button via 4G+; right: IoT temperature, air pressure and motion sensor via 4G+.

A second sensor that also works via NbIoT transmission is a motion-sensitive sensor. This has been installed to register movements in the room and additionally to transmit the room temperature and air pressure to the real-time server via the public radio network. In this case, too, the data is transmitted in JSON format. Further information on the exact key data of the sensors can be found in the publications by Stege et al. [45–48].

2.3.9 Real-time controller

Within the fast care project, the Harz University of Applied Sciences developed a real-time platform for the sensor data fusion of the partial realizations of the partners. For this purpose, a Linux-based application server was configured based on a communication protocol (MQTT) selected for the project. This "real-time controller", on which all information converges, forms the central "sensor data fusion". The device includes a rack mounted server PC with Intel I7 topology and a memory of 16 GByte 1600 MHz DDR3 which is depicted in **Figure 14**. The LINUX version is "Red Hat Enterprise Linux Server release 7.7 (Maipo)". The network interfaces are two 1 GB IEEE 802.3 and a "Realtek Semiconductor Co., Ltd. RTL8192EE PCIe Wireless Network Adapter". More detailed information can be found in [21] the so called final design plan of the fast care project.

2.4 Sensor data visualization

The project partners agreed to the technical implementation of the data fusion on the planned real-time server and the development of a user interface. After the data collection of all partners, these data are evaluated centrally on the real-time controller. The user should receive feedback about the obtained information. This feedback is based on the visualization of the situation analysis. The main view of the

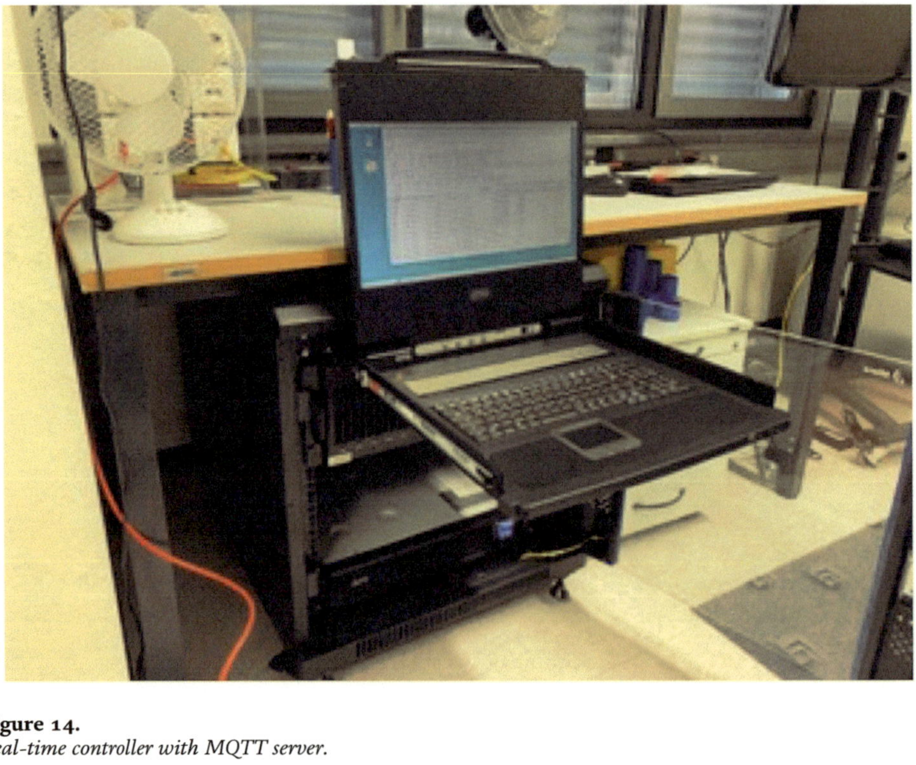

Figure 14.
Real-time controller with MQTT server.

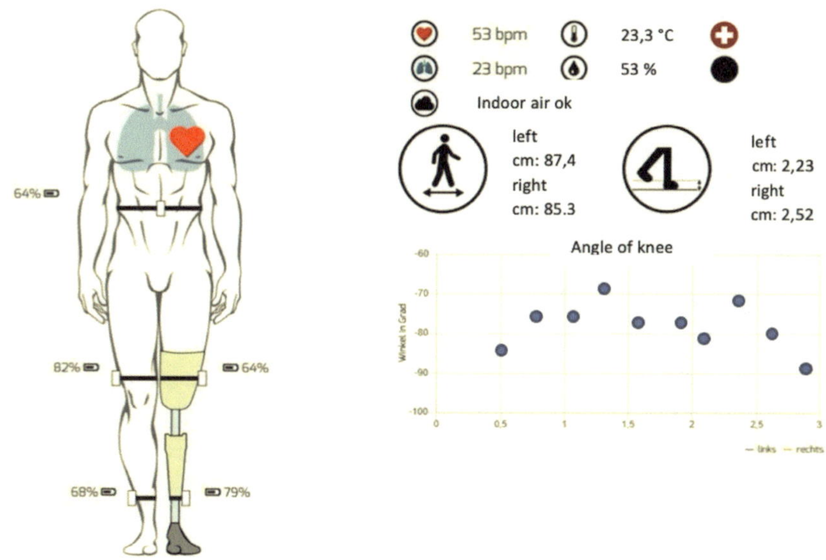

Figure 15.
Real-time visualization of the measured sensor data.

real-time visualization is shown in **Figure 15**. With its end customer platform, Exelonix GmbH forms the technological basis for the visualization in the fast care project. All sensor data collected in the MQTT server of the Harz University of Applied Sciences are evaluated using the Axel Onyx and Customer Platform, and all sensor data collected in the MQTT server of the Harz University are collected using the end customer platform from Exelonix. The sensor data were evaluated and visualized in a web page to which only the project partners had access. The transformation and preparation of the "technical information and data packets" received on the "real-time controller" was realized into a form that can be interpreted by those in need of care, relatives and experts. Among other things, time courses and histories are added.

The visualization is shown in **Figure 15**. An Avatar appears on the left, in which both, the heart rate and the breathing rate are shown optically in a movement of the heart and chest. On the right side of the picture there is a heart with the heart rate and with a lung that the respiratory rate. Furthermore, the data of the Exelonix sensor as well as the emergency button status, the room temperature and the room humidity are shown. An indication of the condition of the indoor air is shown directly below these displays, in this case the icon of a green cloud shows that the indoor air is in good condition.

Additional sensor data is depicted on the Avatar sketch. In the hip, knee and ankle area of the legs, the information about the energetic states of the batteries of the IMUs for recording the posture and knee angle is shown. The measured knee angle from the leg with the prosthesis is shown online in the graphic on the right, where the knee angle is shown in degrees over time while walking.

The measurement of the gait parameters of the patient, which is also recorded by the IMUs on the hips, knees and ankles (see Section 2.3.3), can be seen online to the right of the two icons on the gait width and lifting height of the foot. This allows the gait to be assessed and improved in situ for rehabilitation purposes.

In addition to this main page of the real-time display, a sub-page has been created for each application of the partners, in which the details of the individual sensor elements and their operation are compressed. The details of the real-time visualization of the partners can be seen especially in the final design plan, which can be found in the publication of Kußmann et al. [21].

3. User acceptance studies

In addition to the technical development activities, an analysis of acceptance was executed at the AAL-Lab of the Harz University. As a result of the project, fast care wants to develop feasible products and create the medical fundamentals for an interaction (feedback) in real time.

The project partners agreed to the technical implementation of the data fusion on the planned real-time server and the development of a user interface. This is done in addition to the workload of the integration of all technical components and the planed example application. After the data collection of all partners, these data are evaluated centrally on the real-time controller. The user should receive feedback about the obtained information. This feedback is based on the visualization of the situation analysis.

In the analysis of acceptance of the system, a small sample of a total of 20 subjects from different age groups was interviewed. The following figure shows the distribution by gender and age (**Figure 16**). Although this study is not representative, it gives a first insight into the valuation of the developed technology.

During the survey, the subjects had to assess both the individual systems of the project partners and the overall system. The survey results of the entire system were very positive. 60% of the respondents stated, that they would like to use the technology privately, 70% of the respondents would like to have access to the technology, 35% would be willing to buy the presented technology and 95% see a great benefit for themselves and for others in the tested technology (see **Figure 17**).

In another part of the test, the sample's affinity for technology was queried. On average, the confidence "in your own skills" when dealing with new technology was rated with 3.33 out of 5 points, the willingness to use new and unknown technology with 4 out of 5 points and the degree of technical overload with only 2.13 out of 5 Points. As a result, the test subjects showed a great willingness to use new technologies and did not feel overwhelmed with the used technology (see **Figure 18**).

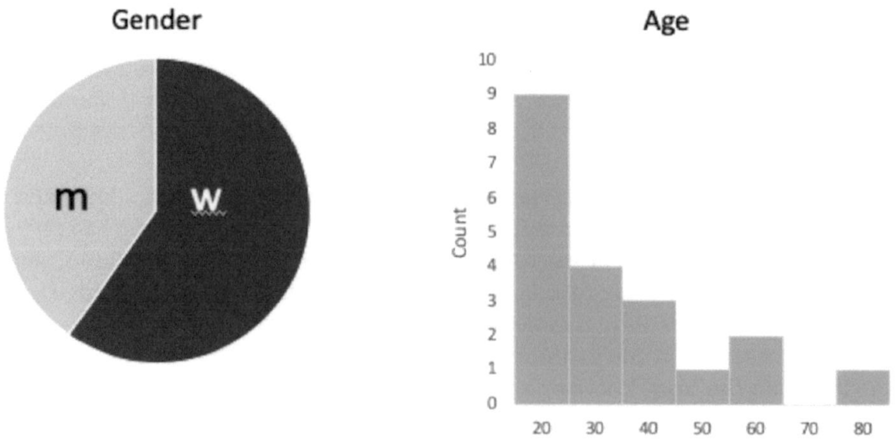

Figure 16.
Age and gender distribution of the testing persons.

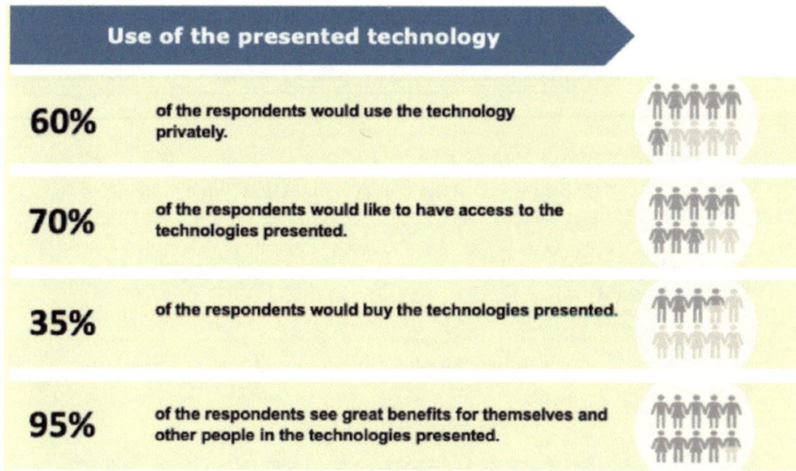

Figure 17.
Use of the presented technologies.

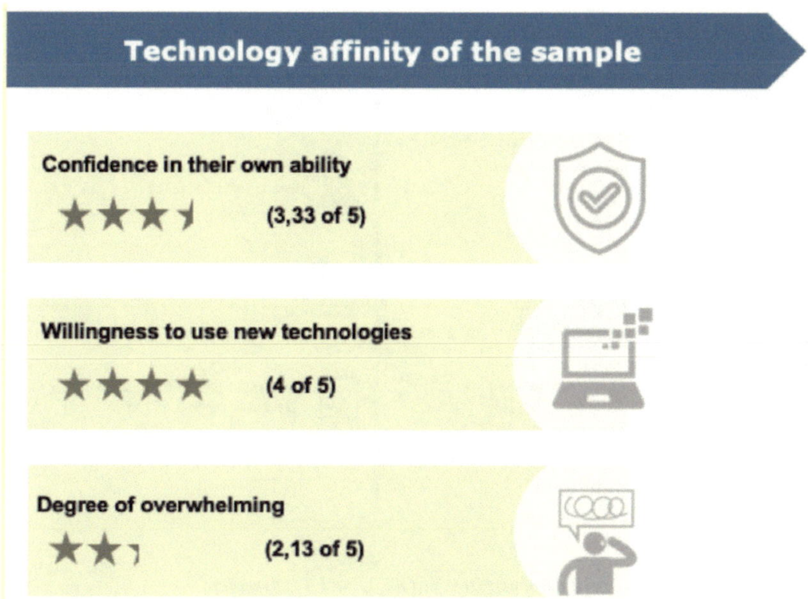

Figure 18.
Technical affinity of the test persons.

Figure 19 illustrates, that the subsystem of the project partner Otto Bock was rated positively by the test subjects. The success of the measurement was rated on average with 4.35 out of 5 points, the success of the calibration with 3.97 out of 5 points and the intelligibility of the display with 3.27 out of 5 points. The women rated the manageability of the system with 4.08 out of 5 points slightly better than the men with 3.44 out of 5 points.

The gait analysis of the project partner of the Otto von Guericke University was rated as very positive by the subjects with 4.27 out of 5 points. The technology used by the OvGU Kinect system with 3.9 out of 5 points. The more the test subjects were overwhelmed with the technology, the more negative the system was rated (see **Figure 20**).

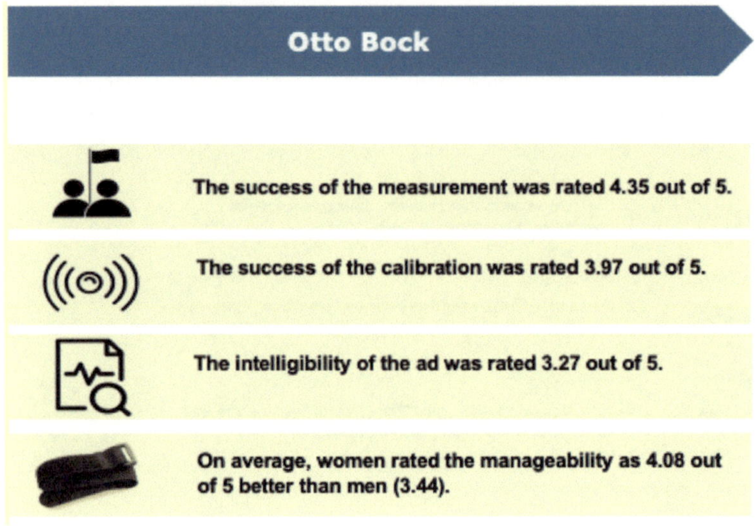

Figure 19.
Evaluation of the application of the active prothetic foot.

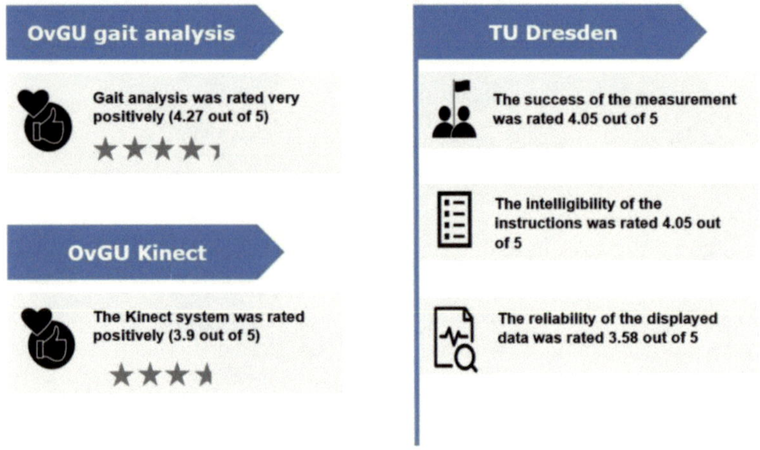

Figure 20.
Evaluation of the applications of the demonstrators of OvGU and TU Dresden.

Analyzing the system of the TU Dresden, the success of the measurement was rated 4.05 out of 5 points and the comprehensibility of the instructions with 4.05 out of 5 points. The comprehensibility of the instructions was more incomprehensible for the test subjects when they were overwhelmed by the technology. The intelligibility of the display and the results was rated with 3.58 out of 5 points (see **Figure 20**).

4. Conclusions

In the project fast care, a real-time capable sensor data analysis-framework in the fields of ambient assisted living was developed. The project realized a medical valid integrated real-time picture of the patient's situation by using several interconnected sensor-actor infrastructures with a latency period of less than 10 ms.

The implemented sensor structure records the heart rate, the breathing rate, the VOC content of the room air, analyzes the gait for rehabilitation and measures the temperature and humidity in the room. An emergency button has also been integrated.

An active prosthetic foot was used as a special application of the sensor-actor System. Its running parameters can be measured online, and the prosthesis can automatically adapt to the floor covering and the running demands via the network. This means that users have an intelligent active prosthesis at their disposal to help them cope with everyday life more easily.

It was shown that even with a heterogeneous network consisting of the components WiFi, Bluetooth LE, Gigabit LAN and 4G+, real-time operation was possible for the use of the AAL components. Even the display of the measured data, which was transferred to a website via the cloud, only showed latencies of an additional few milliseconds. This made it possible to create a real-time image in the form of an Avatar for all vital parameters and the automatic setting of the active prosthetic foot, which enables the client to notice his physical condition in situ.

In addition to the technical development activities, an analysis of acceptance was executed at the demonstrator in the AAL-laboratory. The survey results of the entire system were very positive. 60% of the respondents stated, that they would like to use the technology privately, 70% of the respondents would like to have access to the technology, 35% would be willing to buy the presented technology and 95% see a great benefit for themselves and for others in the tested technology.

Unfortunately, some slow network technologies such as Bluetooth LE had to be used to carry out the project. It is to be expected, that with the full expansion of the networks to the fifth generation (5G), there will still be a significant leap in transmission speed and transmission quality. It is therefore to be expected that eHealth applications in the home area can be implemented in real time in the near future. After the data fusion, further processing with the help of the artificial intelligence will bring further benefits to the client for the prevention of his physical and mental health.

Acknowledgements

The fast care project was supported by the German Federal Ministry of Education and Research in the program “Zwanzig20 – Partnerschaft für Innovation”, contract no. 03ZZ0519I. It was carried out in the form of a joint project with eight partners and a project coordinator. We thank all fast care project partners for their contributions to this work personally listed in the following: Thomas Kirste, Christian Haubelt, Albert Hein, Florian Grützmacher from University Rostock, Ernst Albrecht-Laatsch, Bernhard Graimann, Martin Schmidt and Katharina Olze from Ottobock, Alexander Trumpp, Daniel Wedekind, Martin Schmidt, Sebastian Zaunseder, Hagen Malberg from Technische Universität Dresden, Christian Reinboth and Jens-Uwe Just from HarzOptics, Matthias Stege, Frank Schäfer, Tristan Heinig and Sascha Huth from Exelonix, Rainer Dorsch from Bosch Sensortec, Lutz Schega, Sebastian Stoutz and Kim-Charline Broscheid from Otto-von-Guericke-Universität Magdeburg.

Author details

Ulrich H.P. Fischer*, Sabrina Hoppstock, Peter Kußmann and Isabell Steuding
Harz University of Applied Sciences, Friedrichstr, Wernigerode, Germany

*Address all correspondence to: ufischerhirchert@hs-harz.de

References

[1] Fischer-Hirchert UHP. Anwendung von technikgestützten Pflegeassistenzsystemen in der Harzregion. Geriatric and Gerontology Congress. 2014;**2014**:1

[2] Rost K, Siegmund S, UHP F. Technische Pflegeassistenzsysteme für ein längeres selbstbestimmtes Leben. In: Tagungsband AAL-Konferenz. Berlin: VDE Verlag; 2012. p. 335

[3] Haupt M, Just J-U, Fischer-Hirchert UH. Vitalparametererfassung in technikgestützten Pflegeassistenzsystemen. In: BMC-KONGRESS. Berlin: E.V., Bundesverband Managed Care GGmbH, BMC – Managed Care; 2019. p. 5. Available from: http://www.bmckongress.de

[4] Schelisch L. Wer nutzt eigentlich PAUL? Erfahrungen aus dem Praxiseinsatz. In: VDE (Hrsg.): Wohnen - Pflege - Teilhabe "Besser leben durch Technik". 7. Deutscher AAL- Kongress mit Ausstellung. Elektronische Ressource. Berlin: VDE-Verlag; 21-22 January 2014

[5] Meyer S, Mollenkopf H. In: Coors M, Kumlehn M, editors. Ambient Assisted Living (AAL):Komponenten, Projekte, Services. Eine Bestandsaufnahme. Kohlhammer: Verlag; 2013. p. 220

[6] Kung A, Jean-Bart B. Making AAL platforms a reality. In: Proceedings of the AMI 10 workshop (AmI-10). Ambient Intelligence. Lecture Notes in Computer Science. Vol. 6439. 2010. pp. 187-196

[7] Fischer UHP, Rost K. Businessmodell zur Applikation von AAL-Userportalen zur Verbesserung der sozialen Teilhabe älterer Menschen in der Harzregion. In: AAL-Kongress 2014 Berlin, Wohnen – Pflege – Teilhabe - Besser leben durch Technik. Berlin: VDE; 2014. p. 5

[8] Bauer J, Kettschau, A-K, Franke J. Optimierung der datenvisualisierung von AAL-serviceplattformen durch usability-tests. In: VDE, BMBF, Sozialverband VdK, Fraunhofer-AAL, editors. Wohnen - Pflege - Teilhabe - Besser leben durch Technik. Berlin: VDE Verlag Gmbh; 2014. pp. 1-5

[9] Wagner J, André E, Jung F. Smart sensor integration: A framework for multimodal emotion recognition in real-time. In: Proceedings - 2009 3rd International Conference on Affective Computing and Intelligent Interaction and Workshops. ACII; 2009. p. 2009

[10] Albert M, Görs M, Schilling K. Telemedical applications with rulebased descision- and information-systems (TARDIS). IFAC-PapersOnLine. 2015;**48** (10):7-11. ISSN 2405-8963

[11] Gao W, Emaminejad S, Nyein HYY, Challa S, Chen K, Peck A, et al. Fully integrated wearable sensor arrays for multiplexed in situ perspiration analysis. Nature. January 2016;**28**;529(7587):509-514. DOI: 10.1038/nature16521. PMID: 26819044; PMCID: PMC4996079

[12] Simsek M, Aijaz A, Dohler M, Sachs J, Fettweis G. 5G-enabled tactile internet. IEEE Journal on Selected Areas in Communications. 2016;**34**(3):460-473

[13] Fettweis GP. The tactile internet: Applications and challenges. IEEE Vehicular Technology Magazine. 2014; **9**(1):64-70

[14] Parvez I, Rahmati A, Guvenc I, Sarwat AI, Dai H. A survey on low latency towards 5G: RAN, Core network and caching solutions. IEEE Communication Surveys and Tutorials. 2018;**20**(4):3098-3130

[15] Yao S, Hu S, Zhao Y, Zhang A, Abdelzaher T. DeepSense: A unified deep learning framework for time-series

mobile sensing data processing. In: 26th International World Wide Web Conference. WWW; 2017. p. 2017

[16] Ruhm KH. Sensor fusion and data fusion - mapping and reconstruction. Measurement. 2007;**40**(2):145-157. ISSN 0263-2241. DOI: 10.1016/j.measurement.2006.07.012

[17] Kasetty S, Stafford C, Walker GP, Wang X, Keogh E. Real-time classification of streaming sensor data. In: Proceedings - International Conference on Tools with Artificial Intelligence. ICTAI; 2008

[18] Van Den Bogert AJ, Geijtenbeek T, Even-Zohar O, Steenbrink F, Hardin EC. A real-time system for biomechanical analysis of human movement and muscle function. Medical & Biological Engineering & Computing. October 2013;**51**(10):1069-1077. DOI: 10.1007/s11517-013-1076-z. Epub 2013 Jul 25. PMID: 23884905; PMCID: PMC3751375

[19] mqtt.org. MQTT homepage [Internet]. 2020. Available from: https://mqtt.org

[20] mosquitto.org. MOSQUITTO homepage [Internet]. 2020. Available from: https://www.mosquitto.org

[21] Kußmann P, Hoppstock S, Fischer-Hirchert U. Fast Care Final Design Plan. Wernigerode: Harz University; 2020

[22] Designed by fullvector/Freepik. Server Picture; 2020

[23] Stoutz S, Chen CH, Broscheid KC, Schega L. User acceptance and usability of a home based gait analysis system. In: Smart SysTech 2019 - European Conference on Smart Objects, Systems and Technologies. 2019

[24] Broscheid K-C, SToutz S, Chien-Hsi C, Schega L. The potential of a home-based gait evaluation system with a new low-cost IMU: A pilot study. In: Conference: HEALTH ACROSS LIFESPAN (HAL) - International Conference on Healthiness and Fitness across the Lifespan. Magdeburg: Otto von Guericke University Magdeburg; 12-15-September 2018

[25] Stoutz S, Schega L. Presentation of a concept to support rehabilitation through realtime feedback/monitoring in the home environment. In: Tagung DGBMT. Dresden: VDE; 2017. p. 86. Available from: https://www.vde.com/resource/blob/1645606/36a6dc49966d0b0196c7ddca0c52de8f/bmt2017-dgbmt-jahrestagung-programm-data.pdf

[26] Grützmacher F, Beichler B, Hein A, Kirste T, Haubelt C. Time and memory efficient online piecewise linear approximation of sensor signals. Sensors. 2019;**19**(23):5206

[27] Grützmacher F, Hein A, Kirste T, Haubelt C. Model-based design of energy-efficient human activity recognition systems with wearable sensors. Technology. 2018;**6**(4):89

[28] Hein A, Kirste T. Activity recognition for ambient assisted living: Potential and challenges. Berlin, Germany: Ambient Assisted Living (AAL), Deutscher AAL-Kongress mit Ausstellung / Technologien - Anwendungen - Management; 30 Janauary-01 February 2008. pp. 36-41

[29] Grutzmacher F, Wolff JP, Hein A, Lepidis P, Dorsch R, Kirste T, et al. Towards energy efficient sensor nodes for online activity recognition. In: Proceedings IECON 2017 - 43rd Annual Conference of the IEEE Industrial Electronics Society. 2017

[30] Grützmacher F, Beichler B, Haubelt C. Model-based real time analysis of distributed human activity recognition stages in wireless sensor networks. In: UbiComp/ISWC 2019-Adjunct Proceedings of the 2019 ACM

International Joint Conference on Pervasive and Ubiquitous Computing and Proceedings of the 2019 ACM International Symposium on Wearable Computers. 2019

[31] Hein A, Grützmacher F, Haubelt C, Kirste T. Fast care – Real-time sensor data analysis framework for intelligent assistance systems. Current Directions in Biomedical Engineering. 2017;**3**(2): 743-747

[32] Lempe G, Zaunseder S, Wirthgen T, Zipser S, Malberg H. Kamerabasierte Erfassung kardiorespiratorischer signale. Technisches Messen. 2013;**80**(5):179-184. DOI: 10.1524/teme.2013.0029

[33] Zaunseder S, Heinke A, Trumpp A, Malberg H. Heart beat detection and analysis from videos. In: 2014 IEEE 34th International Scientific Conference on Electronics and Nanotechnology, ELNANO 2014 - Conference Proceedings. 2014

[34] Lempe G, Zaunseder S, Wirthgen T, Zipser S, Malberg H. ROI selection for remote photoplethysmography. In: Meinzer HP, Deserno T, Handels H, Tolxdorff T, editors. Bildverarbeitung für die Medizin. Springer, Berlin, Heidelberg: Informatik aktuell; 2013. Available from: http://doiorg-443.webvpn.fjmu.edu.cn/10.1007/978-3-642-36480-8_19

[35] Takano C, Ohta Y. Heart rate measurement based on a time-lapse image. Medical Engineering & Physics. 2007;**29**(8):853-857

[36] Zaunseder S, Trumpp A, Ernst H, Förster M, Malberg H. Cardiovascular assessment by imaging photoplethysmography – a review. Biomedical Engineering / Biomedizinische Technik. 2018;**63**(5): 617-634. DOI: 10.1515/bmt-2017-0119

[37] Zaunseder S, Trumpp A, Wedekind D, Malberg H. Cardiovascular assessment by imaging photoplethysmography-a review. Biomedizinische Technik. 25 Octobter 2018;**63**(5):617-634. DOI: 10.1515/bmt-2017-0119. PMID: 29897880

[38] Trumpp A, Bauer PL, Rasche S, Malberg H, Zaunseder S. The value of polarization in camera-based photoplethysmography. Biomedical Optics Express. 2017;**8**:2822-2834

[39] Fischer-Hirchert UHP, Reinboth C, Just J-U. Entwicklung von Komponenten für ein verteiltes Sensorsystem zur Echtzeit- Analyse von Atemgas. In: BMC Kongress 2019. Berlin: BMC; 2019. Available from: https://www.bmcev.de/bmc-kongress-posterausstellung/

[40] Khan MRR, Kang B-H, Lee S-W, Kim S-H, Yeom S-H, Lee S-H, et al. Fiber-optic multi-sensor array for detection of low concentration volatile organic compounds. Optics Express. 2013;**21**(17):20119-20130. Available from: http://www.ncbi.nlm.nih.gov/pubmed/24105558

[41] Just J-U, Reinboth C, Kußmann P, Müller A. Realisierung eines Demonstrators zur spektroskopi-schen Analyse von Raumluft und Atemgasen. In: Anhalt H, editor. Nachwuchswissenschaftlerkonferenz. Bernburg: Hochschule Anhalt; 2018. p. 1. Available from: http://nwk2018.de/fileadmin/Dateien/NWK/nwk2018_programmuebersicht.pdf

[42] Khan M, Kang S-W. A high sensitivity and wide dynamic range fiber-optic sensor for low-concentration VOC gas detection. Sensors. 2014; **14**(12):23321-23336. Available from: http://www.mdpi.com/1424-8220/14/12/23321/

[43] Albrecht-laatsch E, Szufnarowski F. Optimization of dynamic properties of exo-prostheses using a distributed inertial measurement system. In:

Jahrestagung der deutschen Gesellschaft für Biomedizinishe Technik DGBMT. Dresden: Saxony; 2017. p. 86. Available from: https://www.vde.com/resource/blob/1645606/36a6dc49966d0b0196c7ddca0c52de8f/bmt2017-dgbmt-jahrestagung-programm-data.pdf

[44] Yordanova K, Hein A, Kirste T. Kitchen Task Assessment Dataset for Measuring Errors Due to Cognitive Impairments. 2020 IEEE International Conference on Pervasive Computing and Communications Workshops (PerCom Workshops), Austin, TX, USA. 2010. pp. 1-6. DOI: 10.1109/PerComWorkshops48775.2020.9156115

[45] Stege M. Requirements of low latency sensor/actuator networks for e-health applications. In: Jahrestagung der BIOMEDIZINISCHEN TECHNIK und Dreiländertagung der MEDIZINISCHEN PHYSIK. Dresden: DGBMT; 2017. p. FS89. Available from: https://www.vde.com/resource/blob/1645606/36a6dc49966d0b0196c7ddca0c52de8f/bmt2017-dgbmt-jahrestagung-programm-data.pdf

[46] Matz AP, Fernandez-Prieto J-A, Cañada-Bago J, Birkel UA. Systematic analysis of narrowband IoT quality of service. Sensors. 2020;**20**:1636-1642

[47] Sunyaev A. The internet of things. In: Internet Computing. Heidelberg: Springer; 2020. DOI: 10.1007/978-3-030-34957-8_10

[48] Exelonix. IoT – Services & Applications E-Health Appications [Internet]. 2020. Available from: https://www.exelonix.com/services_englisch/

Chapter 3

Acoustic Monitoring of Joint Health

Lucy Spain and David Cheneler

Abstract

The joints of the human body, especially the knees, are continually exposed to varying loads as a person goes about their day. These loads may contribute to damage to tissues including cartilage and the development of degenerative medical conditions such as osteoarthritis (OA). The most commonly used method currently for classifying the severity of knee OA is the Kellgren and Lawrence system, whereby a grade (a KL score) from 0 to 4 is determined based on the radiographic evidence. However, radiography cannot directly depict cartilage damage, and there is low inter-observer precision with this method. As such, there has been a significant activity to find non-invasive and radiation-free methods to quantify OA, in order to facilitate the diagnosis and the appropriate course of medical action and to validate the development of therapies in a research or clinical setting. A number of different teams have noted that variation in knee joint sounds during different loading conditions may be indicative of structural changes within the knee potentially linked to OA. Here we will review the use of acoustic methods, such as acoustic Emission (AE) and vibroarthrography (VAG), developed for the monitoring of knee OA, with a focus on the issues surrounding data collection and analysis.

Keywords: ultrasound, acoustic emission, vibroarthrography, osteoarthritis, knee joint

1. Introduction

1.1 Synovial joints and osteoarthritis

The free moving joints within the body are known as synovial joints and have the primary purpose of allowing forces applied to the skeleton to be transmitted as smooth, low-friction movements. The joint capsule, working alongside the muscles, tendons and ligaments stabilises the joint, whilst articular (or hyaline) cartilage covering the end of the bones in combination with synovial fluid within the joint space provides the environment for smooth, well-lubricated movements [1, 2]. In addition, some joints also contain fibrocartilaginous discs between the two bones to support the other joint components and dissipate the forces experienced by the joint, for instance, intervertebral discs in the spine, or the meniscus within the knee.

Osteoarthritis affects all of the structures within the joint and is defined as a condition causing pain within the joint, loss of function and decreased quality of life for patients [3]. The disease results in the degradation of cartilage and subsequent sclerosis and lesions in the now exposed subchondral bone, along with inflammation in the joint [4]. Tears within cartilaginous structures and new

 IntechOpen

interactions between cartilage and bone, along with bone and bone, make for less smooth movements, pain, stiffness and reduction in joint function.

1.2 Epidemiology and impact

The most common joints affected by osteoarthritis include those of the knee, hip and hands with osteoarthritis of the knee the most commonly occurring form, affecting over 18% of the population in England [5].

With such a large proportion of the population affected, musculoskeletal conditions including osteoarthritis have considerable impact both medically and economically. Clinically, the pain and loss of function associated with osteoarthritis result in a lower quality of life reported by patients, who require a large number of GP visits and hospital admissions [6–8].

The underlying pathophysiology of osteoarthritis is unclear, with genetics, age, gender, obesity and previous injury all contributing to varying degrees in disease development and progression. The heterogeneous nature of the disease makes targeted treatment of cause and prevention of progression a challenge, with current best practice centring on patient education and lifestyle changes surrounding exercise, use of analgesics and anti-inflammatories to manage pain and inflammation and finally joint replacement at the severe end of the spectrum of disease [9]. However, this approach, with the exception of exercise targeting weight loss and strength, does not address an underlying cause or prevent progression of disease, an aspiration of future interventions for the disease.

Ranking the sixth most common cause of disability globally in 2010 [10], musculoskeletal conditions, including osteoarthritis, impact not only the healthcare system and patients but also their families [11]. Patients and their carers are at greater risk of being out of employment [12], with only 63% of those with a musculoskeletal condition in employment compared to 82% in those without a health condition [13].

With a predicted increase in the ageing population and an increase in obesity [14–16], the burden on health services and economic impact in terms of lost work time and disability is of growing concern. There is a real need for means of non-invasive early detection of osteoarthritis, sensitive means of monitoring progression and development of efficacious treatments to prevent and improve symptoms in order to improve quality of life and reduce the numbers progressing to severe disease and requiring joint replacement.

2. Standard methods of detection

Osteoarthritis is a condition affecting a multitude of tissues within a joint, and as such, approaches which give information to the clinician on bone, muscle, cartilaginous tissue and the microenvironment within a joint are required to give a full picture of the condition of a joint. Imaging is currently the main diagnostic tool used to assess osteoarthritis. Dependent upon the form of imaging used, a variety of tissues can be examined as markers of disease state and progression.

In clinical practice, a combination of clinical presentation and X-radiography (X-ray) is used to diagnose osteoarthritis. When a patient presents as over 45 years of age, with typical symptoms of osteoarthritis including pain within the joint during activity and minimal stiffness within the joint in the morning lasting no more than 30 min, then X-ray is not indicated for diagnosis [9, 17].

However, X-ray is useful when differential diagnosis is possible, and in certain scenarios, magnetic resonance imaging is used to give additional information on damage to tissues within the joint and inform treatment options.

2.1 X-radiography

X-ray works upon the principle of differential absorbance of radiation by different tissues, with dense tissues such as the bone absorbing a large proportion of the radiation compared to soft tissues such as the muscle and connective tissue.

As a result, the bone appears bright white on images and can be studied for changes in morphology, whereas soft tissues show less differentiation and are not easily examined.

The current gold standard in the diagnosis of osteoarthritis from radiographic images involves the scoring of X-ray images using the Kellgren-Lawrence (KL) scale. The Kellgren-Lawrence is a five-point scale which categorises disease severity based upon the assessment of bony changes, appearances of osteophytes and joint space narrowing within the joint [18]. The description of the radiographic findings at different KL grades can be seen in **Table 1**.

The KL scale was first described in 1957 in response to an identified need to standardise the definition of changes within an osteoarthritic joint in order to improve inter-rater reliability when reporting the disease [18]. Thorough analysis of the performance of the scale at joints throughout the body revealed that whilst correlation between the defined changes and osteoarthritis were observed at all joints bars the wrist, the greatest inter-rater agreement was found within the knee joint. Intra-rater repeatability followed a similar trend with slightly better agreement between readings. This has subsequently been reflected in the most common use of the scale in the assessment of the knee joint.

More recent comparison of radiographic scoring systems has established that for the knee joint, the KL scale has stood the test of time, with no subsequently developed grading systems outperforming the inter-rater repeatability of this scale [19]. However, whilst the limit of inter and intra-observer reliability in assessing radiographic osteoarthritis may have been reached (correlation coefficients around 0.8), it is acknowledged that a more diverse manner of assessment of osteoarthritis may be warranted to improve sensitivity when assessing disease progression and specificity for aspects of the homogeneous pathophysiology underlying the disease.

In terms of sensitivity, KL scoring of radiographs does not perform well in the detection of early disease or in the monitoring of disease progression, where large time periods are required to observe a change in category during which time symptomatic progression may have occurred [20].

Alone, radiographic assessment using the Kellgren-Lawrence scale allows direct assessment of bony changes such as osteophyte formation, however, relies on indirect measures of joint space narrowing to assess cartilaginous change. The surrogate marker of joint space narrowing in place of direct measurement of cartilage, whilst

Grade	Description of radiographic findings
0	No evidence of radiographic osteoarthritis
1	Doubtful narrowing of the joint space and possible osteophytic lipping
2	Definite osteophytes and possible narrowing of the joint space
3	Moderate multiple osteophytes, definite narrowing of the joint space, small pseudocystic areas with sclerotic walls and possible deformity of bone contour
4	Large osteophytes, marked narrowing of joint space, sever sclerosis and definite deformity of bone contour

Table 1.
Kellgren-Lawrence scale description of radiographic findings.

important in the sensitivity of Kellgren-Lawrence scale to disease severity, does not perform well when compared with changes observed arthroscopically [19, 21].

This may go some way to explaining the disparity in patient symptom reporting in the form of self-reported osteoarthritis, clinically diagnosed osteoarthritis and disease severity suggested using the Kellgren-Lawrence scale [22]. In addition to indirect cartilage measurements, the Kellgren-Lawrence score is based solely on the femorotibial joint. As osteoarthritis can also affect the patellofemoral joint, this could account for further disparity between symptoms and radiographic severity of disease [20].

2.2 Magnetic resonance imaging

In contrast to X-radiography, magnetic resonance imaging (MRI) can directly image a number of tissues, including the cartilage, bone and fluids such as that found in the synovium. Several approaches have been taken to the assessment of joints with suspected osteoarthritis using MRI.

A number of joint-specific semi-quantitative scoring systems have been developed using features considered important in osteoarthritis disease manifestation, including bone marrow lesions, meniscal scores and scores of cartilage loss. For the knee, the scoring systems developed include the whole-organ MRI score (WORMS), the knee osteoarthritis scoring system (KOSS), the Boston-Leeds OA knee scoring (BLOKS) and the MRI osteoarthritis knee score (MOAKS), which brings together the strengths of the WORMS and BLOKS systems whilst standardising the definitions used [23].

Quantitative analysis of specific tissues has also been used to measure thickness, area and volume of cartilage, bone area and area of the bone that is denuded, as well as combining the two to assess cartilage thickness over areas of denuded bone. Whilst concentrating on a smaller region of the joint, this approach removes some of the subjectivity associated with the semi-quantitative scores detailed above, both for MRI and X-ray scoring [23–26].

The benefits of MRI for use both clinically and within research are a trade-off between increased sensitivity and specificity and protocols which are realistic for application in a given setting. Semi-quantitative MRI protocols can be performed using clinical MRI equipment, however, have the same caveats of KL scoring of X-rays in terms of inter and intra-rater reliability.

Quantitative measures of the cartilage and bone remove some of the subjective elements of semi-quantitative assessment. The changes of cartilage and bone measurements can be exceedingly small in magnitude, allowing assessment of much smaller anatomical change over shorter timeframes than those observed using X-ray. Making such small measurements presents its own challenges and is time-consuming, whilst producing such small measurements of change that relationship to clinical outcomes can be weak [27]. However, being direct in nature, quantitative measures have shown promise in improving association of imaging techniques with disease symptoms and progression compared with KL scoring of X-rays. Denuded bone area has been shown to correlate with concurrent and incident knee pain [28], whilst changes in cartilage thickness have been linked to the likelihood of disease progression to the point of needing knee joint replacement surgery [29, 30].

In addition to semi-quantitative and quantitative measurements, the use of contrast and powerful MRI imaging protocols extend the means to assess tissue, enabling assessment of components of the ultrastructure of articular cartilage and the meniscus along with the synovial fluid via compositional and diffusion MRI, respectively. This makes MRI a potentially powerful tool in assessing the impact of osteoarthritis on the entirety of a joint, as well as in identifying factors driving disease and predicting disease progression.

High-resolution MRI protocols and high doses of contrast prove most useful in research aimed at understanding of the mechanisms of osteoarthritis and assessment of disease progression or slowing with intervention. However, these are time-consuming protocols and contrast doses can far outstrip recommended doses accepted in clinical practice [31].

The added power of MRI in the assessment of osteoarthritis is most likely to remain predominantly within the research field at this point in time, as access to advanced equipment, lack of uniform protocols and the time-consuming nature of post-processing that is required limits use clinically.

2.3 Other biomarkers of osteoarthritis

Whilst X-Ray and MRI are the two primary forms of imaging used to assess osteoarthritic joints, both computer tomography (CT) and ultrasound have also been employed for this purpose, generally in a research setting, where MRI is proving to provide greatest accuracy [32]. For CT, the use is limited due to CT scans delivering a high radiation dose without delivering significantly greater sensitivity to disease progression than X-ray or MRI.

Whilst ultrasound allows direct imaging of the cartilage which is not obtained during X-ray, interpretation and observations made can vary between operators, especially at joints further from the surface of the skin. This is least marked in superficial joints, and assessment of inflammation and effusion has drawn parallels with disease severity and progression [33–35]. Therefore, ultrasound may be most useful in adding measures associated with inflammation when assessing joints of the hand rather than the knee and hip which are much deeper joints.

Finally, biochemical markers associated with inflammation and degradation of the bone and cartilage are under investigation as additional biomarkers for osteoarthritis. This presents its own challenges as whilst these markers may well be sensitive to change in internal environment, their specificity to osteoarthritis and location of degeneration are proving more of obstacle, with generally weak associations seen between biochemical biomarkers of disease and measures of use in assessing disease severity and progression [36, 37]. That said, there is some evidence that markers may be able to offer additional strength in assessing osteoarthritis severity and response to treatments with further research [38].

2.4 Current challenges in diagnosis and treatment

Individually the current means to diagnose and assess progression of osteoarthritis are limited by one or more factors, namely, subjectivity of measures including high inter- and intra-rater repeatability in semi-quantitative imaging, low sensitivity for change in disease state or low specificity for disease tissue or location.

This presents challenges when making informed clinical decisions, investigating new interventions and determining the effects of preventative measures on disease progression. The low sensitivity of current biomarkers also limits the application of stratified medicine in the approach to new treatments, an area that is of particular interest given the marked clinical and biological heterogeneity of this condition [39].

As the disease is driven by multiple pathogenic factors, it may be that a combination of multiple diagnostic measures is required to develop a sensitive biomarker for osteoarthritis. This concept is currently demonstrated through the development of computational risk factor tools based on a range of self-reported osteoarthritis risk factors, aimed at patient education and pre-emptive lifestyle intervention [40–42]. More recently, the tool for osteoarthritis risk prediction has proven inclusion of MRI measures in combination with KL scored radiographs provides a more powerful predictive tool for predicting disease progression [43]. Furthering this approach using other potential biomarkers for osteoarthritis, including imaging and biochemical markers of cartilage and bone change, may allow even greater sensitivity and specificity.

With this in mind, research has progressed in innovative approaches to develop biosensors that address aspects of osteoarthritis that are currently unmeasured. To date, all biomarkers for the disease consider circulating biochemicals or images of the knee in a static state. As the symptoms of osteoarthritis relate directly to movements of the joint, a novel approach to assessing changes in interactions between tissues during joint movement is being investigated using acoustics within the joint.

3. Acoustic medical technologies for joint health

Due to its non-invasive nature, the use of sound or vibration has found many medical applications associated with the musculoskeletal system.

For instance, as discussed above, ultrasound imaging, or ultrasonography (US), can be a useful tool in rheumatology. It is increasingly used to image and evaluate the inflammatory aspects of rheumatic diseases as an assessment tool for tendons and soft tissue [44, 45]. It has been applied to osteoarthritis specifically, having been shown to be a sensitive tool for the evaluation of synovitis (joint inflammation) and joint effusion (the flow of blood and other fluids in joints), through direct imaging and the use of Doppler signal analysis, a form of flow velocimetry [44–48]. Whilst US can be used for imaging musculoskeletal changes in osteoarthritis, such as changes in cartilage thickness, it is limited. It has been noted that US may be limited in assessing cartilage in larger weight-bearing joints [49] because of the inherent inability of ultrasound to pass through denser bony structures and therefore penetrate to the deeper portions of the joint [50]. The central portion of thick joints cannot be visualised with US [51], but US can detect osteophytosis (bone spurs forming around joints) at greater rates than conventional radiography. Being non-ionising and able to image soft tissues, US is a good alternative to radiographic imaging. Magnetic resonance imaging (MRI) offers excellent tissue contrast and anatomical resolution compared to US [49]. MRI can detect changes in the volumes of cartilage, whereas US is only capable of quantifying changes in thicknesses. Therefore, whilst MRI is more expensive, US is primarily only used as an alternative for anatomical imaging when there is hardware present within the patient, i.e. implants and some older cardiac defibrillators and pacemakers, which precludes the use of MRI [52].

As well as for imaging, ultrasound can be utilised directly as a treatment for OA [53, 54]. The management of OA involves the relief of pain and the maintenance or improvement of joint function. The American College of Rheumatology (ACR) and the European League Against Rheumatism (EULAR) recommend a combination of pharmacological and nonpharmacological treatments [55]. Various nonpharmacological treatments, including exercise, physical therapy, hot packs and therapeutic ultrasound (TU) etc., exist with varying evidence of efficacy. In TU, mechanical energy in the form of pulsed or continuous high-frequency vibrations is applied directly to the joint [56]. This is reputed to reduce oedema or cysts [57], as well as reduce inflammation, relieve pain and accelerate tissue repair; however, results of clinical studies are conflicting [55, 56]. The applied ultrasonic vibrations cause atomic oscillations in the tissue; the amplitude of which depends on the intensity or power of the applied beam. When applied continuously, this can result in thermal effects in the tissue, which are reduced when the beam is pulsed [56]. When the ultrasonic beam has high intensity, the atoms in the attenuating medium no longer oscillate around their equilibrium position but have a net motion along the axis of the beam [53]. This can result in damage or micro-machining due to the ultrasound-induced forces, allowing TU to be used as a surgical tool [53]. High-intensity TU can also result in the movement of particles and fluid within the tissue. This phenomenon has been used to drive pharmaceuticals, such as non-steroidal anti-inflammatory drugs (NSAIDs) and corticosteroids, into the tissue [58, 59], facilitating local delivery.

3.1 Acoustic detection

Spontaneous emission of acoustic waves and other vibrations has been recorded during the flexion and extension of joints, as well as the fracture and wear of bones and implants [60, 61]. Studies have shown that these vibrations are affected by musculoskeletal disorders in joints, making vibration monitoring a useful diagnostic tool [62]. However, joints are highly complex heterogeneous structures over a wide range of length scales. Parameters like wave velocity, dispersion and attenuation all affect how waves travel through tissues, making interpretation of the waveform complicated. The following techniques have been developed to resolve this issue:

3.1.1 Phonoarthrography

The earliest studies on the monitoring of the spontaneous emission of acoustic waves were based on the use of stethoscopes to amplify audible sounds generated within joints [63, 64]. Early joint auscultation in this manner was initially a manual process and was inherently subjective. Still, these studies showed that whilst there are 'normal joint sounds', the sound produced is affected by different kinds of injury and arthritis [65]. That said, this method is not yet used in primary care and has only received modest attention in the literature since its first appearance in 1902 [63, 66].

Later studies attempted to reduce the subjectivity of this method by recording the sounds using microphones in conjunction with joint measurement technologies such as goniometers and video tracking [67]. Several of these studies note that pathological signals have major frequency components at low frequencies, that is, below 1000 Hz [64, 68]. The sensitivity range of the microphones used is usually in the range 50 Hz to 15 kHz; however, it has been suggested that standard acoustic recording microphones are not appropriate for the monitoring of joint signals, being too sensitive to background noise, with vibration transducers, or contact sensors, and accelerometers being preferred [61, 69]. Studies such as that by Chu et al. employed a differential microphone pair for noise cancellation and bandpass filters to minimise low-frequency movement artefacts and high-frequency transducer noise to mitigate this issue [61]. Conversely, other studies [70] suggest that as microphones are able to detect higher frequencies and no direct contact with the body is required, the combination of signals from both microphones and accelerometers might perform better than anyone signal alone.

Data analysis in early studies generally only used traditional stationary spectrum estimation methods using oscilloscopes or narrow-band spectrum analysers, with key measures being the frequency, wavelength, wave number and amplitude [64]. However, it is clear that the signals are nonstationary in nature, especially as different signals are generated at different joint positions [69]. As a result of this observation, more sophisticated spectral analysis methods were developed. One method is short-time Fourier analysis on segmented data where it is assumed that the data is stationary within each segment. This allows trends in the frequency component of the signal to be correlated with joint angle. The determination of the segments introduces subjectivity into the analysis. Therefore, techniques to track the nonstationarities in the signal, such as adaptive segmentation, linear prediction and autoregressive moving averages (ARMA), have been incorporated into the analysis [69].

3.1.2 Vibroarthrography (VAG)

Whilst phonoarthrography is based on the sound produced during the flexion or extension of joints, in VAG all vibrations produced during movement are considered [62]. Consequently, it is more common for a single accelerometer to be used as the sensor rather than a microphone [71]. It is also very common for signals in a frequency range below 1000 Hz to be of primary focus [72], with sampling rates of the order 1–4 kHz. A key advantage of the low sampling rate is that it allows for wireless data acquisition and processing using simple microcontrollers or single-board computers [73, 74]. That said, it has been suggested [71, 75] that single signal processing may be limited and multi-channel recordings may lead to better discrimination of the severity and location of joint injury or disorder. In many cases noise mitigation is achieved through prefiltering (commonly using a bandpass filter from 10 Hz to 1 kHz) and amplification prior to digitization at a specified sampling rate [76, 77]. The digital signal may go through additional filtering, such as that conducted by Andersen et al. [78] who used a Kaiser-windowed finite impulse response (FIR) bandpass filter.

There are other rationales for using multiple sensors during VAG as it has been observed that VAG may pick up vibrations not necessarily just due to the joint directly or to external interference [79]. For instance, the 10 Hz signal generated by the rectus femoris muscle which activates during the extension of the leg could interfere with the VAG signal recorded from the skin surface over the patella [80]. As this signal may vary in a similar fashion to the VAG signal, simple bandpass filtering may not be sufficient. It may be necessary to record the vibromyogram at the rectus femoris at the same time as the VAG signal and use adaptive filtering and noise cancellation techniques to isolate the VAG signal [79].

Therefore, the VAG signal is inherently nonstationary and potentially multicomponent in nature. The nature of the VAG signal means that it is not easily analysed using common signal processing techniques. This coupled with the difficulty in ascertaining the biological origin of the source of the signal is the main barrier to its use as a common diagnostic tool. As a result, much of the recent research activity has been focussed on feature extraction and statistical pattern classification [60]. Adaptive segmentation using least-square, linear prediction and autoregression algorithms is common [81, 82]. A host of statistical measures has been considered to characterise the VAG signal, including the form factors, skewness, kurtosis and entropy [71, 76]. It has also been shown that time-frequency distribution (TFD) [81, 83] and wavelet decomposition [84] are potentially powerful techniques for analysis and may negate the need for segmentation [83] but may be susceptible to noise [85]. These advancements have mostly been driven by developments in digital signal processing technologies that sped up analysis time as well as nonstationary signal analysis techniques developed for other biological signals like EEGs [84].

Using these techniques, spectral features such as frequency, energy and their respective spreads can be classified and linked to joint position, loading and pathology. The commonly used classifiers are neural network-based classifiers and support vector machines (SVM), as well as logistic regression and rule-based techniques [62, 71]. These neural networks and SVMs are supervised learning algorithms which search for a number of independent training data patterns taken from signals measured from participants with known pathologies to characterise new signals. These classification algorithms are increasingly dependable and can perform well with a limited amount of data. A number of different variants of these algorithms and classifiers have been investigated [60, 62]. Wu et al. [73] used an SVM based on the entropy and envelope amplitude features and achieved an overall accuracy of 83.56%. Nalband et al. [86] utilised an a priori algorithm with a least-square SVM classifier and claim accuracy of 94.31% with a false discovery rate of 0.0892. Kręcisz [87] achieved accuracies of >90% using a logistic regression-based method. In each of these cases, the VAG signals were collected during knee flexion/extension motion using an accelerometer secured to the participants patella.

3.1.3 Acoustic emission (AE)

AE for biomedical applications is derived from non-destructive techniques developed for detecting damage in engineering materials, such as metals and composites [88]. AE occurs when materials locally under stress emit energy in the form of transient elastic waves. This allows for the monitoring of microcrack initiation and propagation in the bones and joints [89]—essential parts of bone remodelling [90], and wear [91, 92]. Other characteristic sounds in joints, such as the bursting of gas bubbles in synovial joints during movement, can also be detected using AE [93]. AE frequencies are usually in the ultrasonic range and so detection often involves the use of ultrasonic sensors.

A number of researchers have proposed AE sensor-based joint monitoring systems using piezoelectric films, electret or MEMS-based microphones.

Toreyin et al. [94, 95] used an off-the-shelf low-noise MEMS microphone in conjunction with gyroscope and accelerometer pairs in order to monitor sounds generated during various complex motions. The microphone used had a sensitivity range of 100 Hz to 10 kHz, and the researchers suggested that the MEMS-based microphone had a similar performance to an electret microphone [94]. The acoustic data were sampled at 100 kHz, and the inertial data (monitoring joint angle and limb movement) at 1 kHz, with the data being collected by a field programmable gate array (FPGA)-based real-time processor. It was noted that air microphones do not exhibit signal losses due to motion artefacts, but they are sensitive to ambient noise.

Teague et al. [96] compared a piezoelectric film-based contact microphone to two air microphones: one electret and one MEMS-based. The air microphones were used with a 15 Hz high-pass filter and a second-order low-pass filter with a cut-off frequency of 21 kHz and sampled at 44.1 kHz using an acoustic recorder. The piezoelectric microphone was used with a 100 Hz high-pass filter followed by a fourth order low-pass filter with a 10 kHz cut-off frequency. It was sampled at 50 kHz using custom circuits. The 100 Hz high-pass filter was chosen to attenuate the motion artefact noise. It was noted that the electret and MEMS microphones performed similarly in detecting joint sounds, although the electret sensor was significantly more expensive. They were both sensitive to ambient and interface noise, including rubbing of the tape securing the sensors. It was noted that the air microphones did not need to be in contact with the skin. Experiments with sensors positioned 5 cm off the skin captured similar acoustic signals, albeit with lower amplitude. The piezoelectric sensor was more sensitive to interface noise but less sensitive to background noise. Importantly, the contact microphone did not pick up higher frequency vibrations as distinctly as the air microphones which provided higher quality recordings as indicated by higher SNIRs.

Jeong et al. [97] used a low-noise electret microphone with a frequency range of 50 Hz to 20 kHz recorded by an audio recorder at a rate of 44.1 kHz. Signals were digitally filtered using a finite impulse response bandpass filter with a bandwidth from 1 to 15 kHz to prioritise short duration joint sounds whilst supressing interface noise.

Feng and Chen [98] developed a piezoelectric sensor comprised of a lead zirconium titanate (PZT) film deposited on titanium cantilever arrays as an acoustic sensing layer. This sensor uses a 1-mm-tall SU8 cylindrical probe on each cantilever to be in direct contact with the skin of the participant and transmit vibrations to the sensor. A thermoresponsive poly(N-isopropylacrylamide) (PNIPA) film was integrated into the sensor to apply a force to the cantilever and hence improve contact between the probe and the skin when a current is applied across it. The sensor achieved a frequency range of up to 100 kHz, with at least one strong resonant peak at 390 Hz. A sampling rate of 2 MHz was used with a 1 kHz high-pass digital filter to remove low-frequency noise signals. Testing of the sensor on a butchered porcine leg during repeated joint flexure cycles revealed the presence of well-defined peaks located between 30 and 40 kHz, 60 and 70 kHz and 70 and 80 kHz. Similar trends to that observed with commercial AE sensors (the same used in the studies by Mascaro et al. in the JAAS system described later [99]) were noted during overuse of the joint.

Choi et al. [93] developed the bone joint acoustic sensor (BJAS). This has a pin-type probe on a disk-shaped piezoceramic supported by a damped metal plate. The structure is in a metal case with the probe in direct contact with the skin. The system used in conjunction with IMUs seems to have a frequency range of 100 Hz to 25 kHz and is sampled at 50 kHz.

Shark and Goodacre developed the joint acoustic analysis system (JAAS) [99, 100]. This system uses commercial piezoelectric contact ultrasonic acoustic sensors (with high sensitivity in the range 50–200 kHz but monitored over 20–400 kHz at a 1–5 MSPS sampling rate) [100] and electro-goniometers to provide joint angle-based AE during knee joint movement (see **Figure 1**). These commercial AE sensors use relatively thick piezoelectric bulk blocks for AE sensing and are housed in metal shells. The housing is fixed to the skin with surgical tape to maintain a rigid contact. The AE data acquisition operates in a non-continuous recording mode to minimise data volume. When the AE PCI data acquisition board is triggered by a signal value above a pre-set threshold, a 'hit' is recorded corresponding to an acoustic event. Each AE hit is recorded with a set of characteristic waveform features (i.e. dominant frequency, maximum amplitude and duration), and in addition the full waveforms were also stored, digitalized at a 1 MHz sampling frequency over a maximum duration of 15 ms [99]. The number of hits during each joint motion was used to determine a correlation with OA severity defined by KL scores determined using MRI data. It was noted that the frequency response of the acoustic sensor data is characterised by two peaks with a high probability of occurrence during

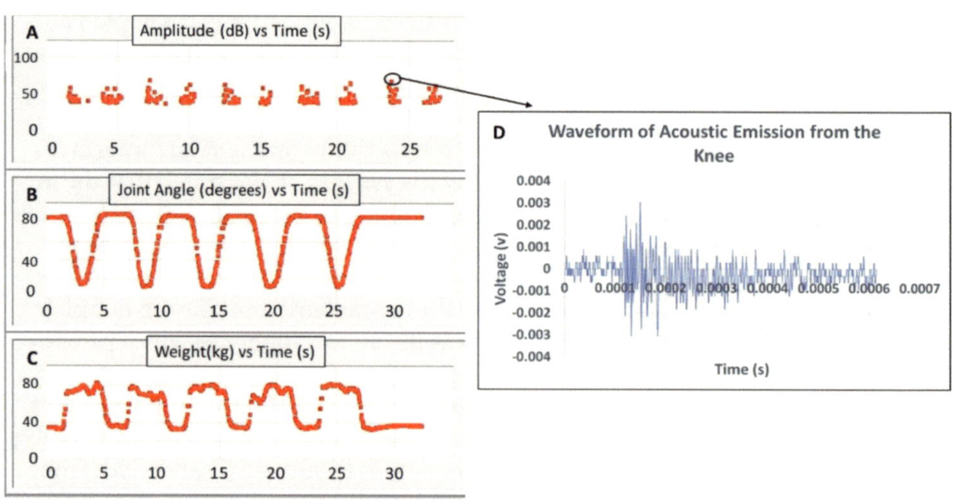

Figure 1.
Output from the joint acoustic analysis system (JAAS). Recording is made as the participant performs five sit-stand-sit movements. A: Acoustic 'hits' from a single knee recorded using a piezoelectric contact ultrasonic acoustic sensors. Each square indicates one acoustic emission captured by the system. For each 'hit' a waveform is also captured [D] from which waveform characteristics are calculated by the software. Alongside the acoustic emissions, joint angle [B] and weight through the leg [C] are also recorded.

knee measurements using a sit-stand-sit protocol, one in the low-frequency range (20–50 kHz) and the other one around 150 kHz. The latter frequency is mainly due to a peak of sensitivity of the sensor used [99].

4. Conclusion

Using radiographic techniques to monitor variations in joint structure and morphology is the classic method of quantifying OA. However, this technique is ionising, often requires multiple measurements as only the plane perpendicular to the radiation is observed and cannot monitor soft tissue directly. MRI can measure the thickness and volume of cartilage, but there are limitations with respect to time and cost. Ultrasound can monitor joint effusion and the thickness of cartilage, but it is not possible for ultrasound to penetrate thick bone tissue and observe the whole joint. There is the additional issue of subjectivity and the large difference in reproducibility based on the skill of those analysing the image. The use of invasive cameras in arthroscopy and joint endoscopy necessitate recovery after diagnosis. These techniques also do not facilitate measurements using dynamic movements. The use of acoustic sensors has the potential to quantify and classify joint pathology whilst removing the subjectivity of classic imaging techniques. Despite progress in detecting differences between type and severity of joint disorders, questions remain about the true origin and form of acoustic signals generated by joint structural changes. Thus, a significant part of the challenge linked to acoustic signal analysis resides in the retrieval of pertinent parameters from irrelevant information in a robust and statistically significant way [78].

As yet, whilst several protocols, sensor types and data analysis techniques have been developed, to date there is no consensus on the most adequate way to record and process vibration data [60]. The methodological aspects of acoustic assessments, such as sensor placement and outcomes measures have not been thoroughly investigated allowing doubt in the technique to remain. For instance, for knee investigations, many studies [73, 81, 101] favour what may be called an open kinematic chain configuration [102] whereby participants sit in a chair and lift their legs in a repetitive fashion, perhaps with weights attached. This has the advantage of being able to vary the load on the joint and allow for the inclusion of participants with advanced degenerative conditions or injuries affecting the limitation of the range of motion in the joint. A common alternative protocol involves repeated sit-stand-sit movements [103–105], creating a closed kinematic chain. This latter configuration perhaps has the advantage of forming a more natural loading of the knee joint. It potentially has the consequence of being inconsistent over time, as people can have the tendency of adjusting their movement to compensate for restricted or painful movement, thus changing the distribution of forces and moments acting on the knee [106]. Data comparing the protocols is limited, and there is no strong evidence for favouring one protocol over the other or indeed over alternatives, such as squatting [94, 102]. Given the protocol affects the loading of the joint and the frequency response of the vibration data generated, it also affects the potential consistency of the statistics derived therefrom and their subsequent interpretation for diagnostic and prognostic purposes. This suggests the necessity of a standard protocol if such techniques are to be used for monitoring the development of OA in an individual over time for clinical or research purposes.

Similarly, it is unclear what sort of vibrations and which frequency range is the most pertinent range to measure. In phonoarthrography acoustic waves in the audible range are of most interest. In VAG, focus is on low-frequency (<1000 Hz) vibrations, the cause and nature of which is more general. In AE, acoustic signals are of primary focus, albeit generally of a higher frequency than that used in phonoarthrography. Whilst there is a significant amount of overlap between the techniques, there are important data that can be missed if one technique is favoured. There is little evidence to suggest that one technique is inherently better than the other, simply due to the lack of comparative studies. The lack of commonality in technique makes meta-analysis difficult. One limitation that is preventing the direct comparison is the lack of technologies that allow high-quality acoustic data to be collected at high sampling rates (>5 MSPS) for significant time periods as such sensors will inherently generate vast amounts of data requiring significant processing. Multiple sensors covering the different frequency ranges of interest are likely to be the way forward, but this strategy will have the disadvantage of comparing signals recorded at different sites, making the analysis more difficult. In any case, further study relating the acoustic signal back to the biomechanics of joint pathology may provide a stronger scientific basis to the causation of the signal, instead of relying on correlations. This will reduce the subjectivity of the analysis and facilitate diagnosis and prognosis, allowing this technique to become a powerful clinical tool.

Acknowledgements

We thank the research team at Lancaster University, led by Prof. Goodacre, who helped in the development of the concepts within this chapter. We also thank the University of Cumbria for providing funding to support the publication of this chapter.

Conflict of interest

The authors declare that they have no conflict of interest.

Author details

Lucy Spain[1] and David Cheneler[2]*

1 University of Cumbria, Carlisle, UK

2 Engineering, Lancaster University, Lancaster, UK

*Address all correspondence to: d.cheneler@lancaster.ac.uk

References

[1] Drake R, Vogl AW, Mitchell AWM. Gray's Anatomy for Students. 2nd ed. Philadelphia, USA: Elsevier Health Sciences; 2009. pp. 1103

[2] Martin RB, Burr DB, Sharkey NA, Fyhrie DP. Synovial joint mechanics. In: Martin RB, Burr DB, Sharkey NA, Fyhrie DP, editors. Skeletal Tissue Mechanics [Internet]. New York, NY: Springer; 2015. pp. 227-273. DOI: 10.1007/978-1-4939-3002-9_5

[3] National Collaborating Centre for Chronic Conditions. Osteoarthritis: National clinical guideline for care and management in adults. London: Royal College of Physicians; 2008

[4] Man G, Mologhianu G. Osteoarthritis pathogenesis—A complex process that involves the entire joint. Journal of Medicine and Life. 2014;7(1):37-41

[5] Public Health England. Public Health Profiles © Crown copyright. 2020 [Internet]. Available from: https://fingertips.phe.org.uk

[6] Arthritis Research UK National Primary Care Centre. Musculoskeletal Matters: Bulletin 2. Keele University: Arthritis Research UK National Primary Care Centre; 2009

[7] Dominick KL, Ahern FM, Gold CH, Heller DA. Health-related quality of life and health service use among older adults with osteoarthritis. Arthritis Care & Research. 2004;**51**(3):326-331

[8] NHS Digital. Hospital Admitted Patient Care and Adult Critical Care Activity 2017-2018. NHS Digital; 2018

[9] NICE. Osteoarthritis: Care and management [Internet]. National Institute for Health and Care Excellence; 2014. Available from: https://www.nice.org.uk/guidance/cg177/chapter/1-Recommendations#education-and-self-management-2

[10] Vos T, Flaxman AD, Naghavi M, Lozano R, Michaud C, Ezzati M, et al. Years lived with disability (YLDs) for 1160 sequelae of 289 diseases and injuries 1990-2010: A systematic analysis for the Global Burden of Disease Study 2010. Lancet London England. 2012;**380**(9859):2163-2196

[11] Dueñas M, Ojeda B, Salazar A, Mico JA, Failde I. A review of chronic pain impact on patients, their social environment and the health care system. Journal of Pain Research. 2016;**9**:457-467

[12] Marmot M, Goldblatt P, Allen J. Fair Society, Healthy Lives: Strategic Review of Health Inequalities. London: The Marmot Review Team; 2010

[13] Office for National Statistics. Labour force survey: Performance and quality monitoring report, April to June 2017 [Internet]. 2017. Available from: https://www.ons.gov.uk/employmentandlabourmarket/peopleinwork/employmentandemployeetypes/methodologies/labourforcesurveyperformanceandqualitymonitoringreports/labourforcesurveyperformanceandqualitymonitoringreportapriltojune2017

[14] National Academies of Sciences E, Division of Health and Medicine, Board of Food and Nutrition, Roundtable on Obesity, Callahan EA. Current Status and Response to the Global Obesity Pandemic: Proceedings of a Workshop [Internet]. Washington, DC: National Academies Press (US); 2019. Available from: https://www.ncbi.nlm.nih.gov/books/NBK544130/

[15] Office for National Statistics. Estimates of the very old, including centenarians, UK [Internet]. 2018. Available from: https://www.ons.gov.uk/peoplepopulationandcommunity/birthsdeathsandmarriages/ageing/

bulletins/estimatesoftheveryoldincludingcentenarians/2002to2018

[16] United Nations, DESA, Population Division. World Population Prospects [Internet]. 2019. Available from: https://population.un.org/wpp/

[17] Sakellariou G, Conaghan PG, Zhang W, Bijlsma JWJ, Boyesen P, D'Agostino MA, et al. EULAR recommendations for the use of imaging in the clinical management of peripheral joint osteoarthritis. Annals of the Rheumatic Diseases. 2017;**76**(9):1484-1494

[18] Kellgren JH, Lawrence JS. Radiological assessment of osteo-arthrosis. Annals of the Rheumatic Diseases. 1957;**16**(4):494-502

[19] Wright RW, MARS Group. Osteoarthritis classification scales: Interobserver reliability and arthroscopic correlation. Journal of Bone and Joint Surgery. 2014;**96**(14):1145-1151

[20] Kohn MD, Sassoon AA, Fernando ND. Classifications in brief: Kellgren-Lawrence classification of osteoarthritis. Clinical Orthopaedics and Related Research. 2016;**474**(8):1886-1893

[21] Kijowski R, Blankenbaker D, Stanton P, Fine J, De Smet A. Arthroscopic validation of radiographic grading scales of osteoarthritis of the tibiofemoral joint. American Journal of Roentgenology. 2006;**187**(3):794-799

[22] Parsons C, Clynes M, Syddall H, Jagannath D, Litwic A, van der Pas S, et al. How well do radiographic, clinical and self-reported diagnoses of knee osteoarthritis agree? Findings from the Hertfordshire cohort study. SpringerPlus. 2015;**4**(1):177

[23] Hunter DJ, Guermazi A, Lo GH, Grainger AJ, Conaghan PG, Boudreau RM, et al. Evolution of semi-quantitative whole joint assessment of knee OA: MOAKS (MRI Osteoarthritis Knee Score). Osteoarthritis Cartilage. 2011;**19**(8):990-1002

[24] Hunter DJ, Lo GH, Gale D, Grainger AJ, Guermazi A, Conaghan PG. The reliability of a new scoring system for knee osteoarthritis MRI and the validity of bone marrow lesion assessment: BLOKS (Boston Leeds Osteoarthritis Knee Score). Annals of the Rheumatic Diseases. 2008;**67**(2):206-211

[25] Kornaat PR, Ceulemans RYT, Kroon HM, Riyazi N, Kloppenburg M, Carter WO, et al. MRI assessment of knee osteoarthritis: Knee Osteoarthritis Scoring System (KOSS)—Inter-observer and intra-observer reproducibility of a compartment-based scoring system. Skeletal Radiology. 2005;**34**(2):95-102

[26] Peterfy CG, Guermazi A, Zaim S, Tirman PFJ, Miaux Y, White D, et al. Whole-Organ Magnetic Resonance Imaging Score (WORMS) of the knee in osteoarthritis. Osteoarthritis Cartilage. 2004;**12**(3):177-190

[27] Spain L, Rajoub B, Schlüter DK, Waterton JC, Bowes MA, Shark L-K, et al. Biomarkers for knee osteoarthritis: New technologies, new paradigms. 2015

[28] Cotofana S, Wyman BT, Benichou O, Dreher D, Nevitt M, Gardiner J, et al. Relationship between knee pain and the presence, location, size and phenotype of femorotibial denuded areas of subchondral bone as visualized by MRI. Osteoarthritis Cartilage. 2013;**21**(9):1214-1222

[29] Eckstein F, Kwoh CK, Boudreau RM, Wang Z, Hannon MJ, Cotofana S, et al. Quantitative MRI measures of cartilage predict knee replacement: A case-control study from the Osteoarthritis Initiative. Annals of the Rheumatic Diseases. 2013;**72**(5):707-714

[30] Pelletier J-P, Cooper C, Peterfy C, Reginster J-Y, Brandi M-L, Bruyère O, et al. What is the predictive value of MRI for the occurrence of knee replacement surgery in knee osteoarthritis? Annals of the Rheumatic Diseases. 2013;**72**(10):1594-1604

[31] Li Q, Amano K, Link TM, Ma CB. Advanced imaging in osteoarthritis. Sports Health. 2016;**8**(5):418-428

[32] Chan WP, Lang P, Stevens MP, Sack K, Majumdar S, Stoller DW, et al. Osteoarthritis of the knee: Comparison of radiography, CT, and MR imaging to assess extent and severity. American Journal of Roentgenology. 1991;**157**(4):799-806

[33] Conaghan PG, D'Agostino MA, Le Bars M, Baron G, Schmidely N, Wakefield R, et al. Clinical and ultrasonographic predictors of joint replacement for knee osteoarthritis: Results from a large, 3-year, prospective EULAR study. Annals of the Rheumatic Diseases. 2010;**69**(4):644-647

[34] Mancarella L, Addimanda O, Pelotti P, Pignotti E, Pulsatelli L, Meliconi R. Ultrasound detected inflammation is associated with the development of new bone erosions in hand osteoarthritis: A longitudinal study over 3.9 years. Osteoarthritis Cartilage. 2015;**23**(11):1925-1932

[35] Mathiessen A, Slatkowsky-Christensen B, Kvien TK, Hammer HB, Haugen IK. Ultrasound-detected inflammation predicts radiographic progression in hand osteoarthritis after 5 years. Annals of the Rheumatic Diseases. 2016;**75**(5):825-830

[36] Deveza LA, Kraus VB, Collins JE, Guermazi A, Roemer FW, Bowes M, et al. Association between biochemical markers of bone turnover and bone changes on imaging: Data from the osteoarthritis initiative. Arthritis Care & Research. 2017;**69**(8):1179-1191

[37] Lotz M, Martel-Pelletier J, Christiansen C, Brandi M-L, Bruyère O, Chapurlat R, et al. Republished: Value of biomarkers in osteoarthritis: Current status and perspectives. Postgraduate Medical Journal. 2014;**90**(1061):171-178

[38] Sofat N, Ejindu V, Heron C, Harrison A, Koushesh S, Assi L, et al. Biomarkers in painful symptomatic knee OA demonstrate that MRI assessed joint damage and type II collagen degradation products are linked to disease progression. Frontiers in Neuroscience. 2019;**13**:1016. Available from: https://www.frontiersin.org/articles/10.3389/fnins.2019.01016/full

[39] Mimpen JY, Snelling SJB. Chondroprotective factors in osteoarthritis: A joint affair. Current Rheumatology Reports. 2019;**21**(8):41. Available from: https://www.ncbi.nlm.nih.gov/pmc/articles/PMC6588640/

[40] Losina E, Michl GL, Smith KC, Katz JN. Randomized controlled trial of an educational intervention using an online risk calculator for knee osteoarthritis: Effect on risk perception. Arthritis Care & Research. 2017;**69**(8):1164-1170

[41] Losina E, Klara K, Michl GL, Collins JE, Katz JN. Development and feasibility of a personalized, interactive risk calculator for knee osteoarthritis. BMC Musculoskeletal Disorders. 2015;**16**(1):312

[42] Yoo TK, Kim DW, Choi SB, Oh E, Park JS. Simple scoring system and artificial neural network for knee osteoarthritis risk prediction: A cross-sectional study. PLoS ONE. 2016;**11**(2):e0148724

[43] Joseph GB, McCulloch CE, Nevitt MC, Neumann J, Gersing AS, Kretzschmar M, et al. Tool for osteoarthritis risk prediction (TOARP) over 8 years using baseline clinical data, X-ray, and MR imaging—Data from

the Osteoarthritis Initiative. Journal of Magnetic Resonance Imaging. 2018;**47**(6):1517-1526

[44] Iagnocco A. Imaging the joint in osteoarthritis: A place for ultrasound? Best Practice & Research: Clinical Rheumatology. 2010;**24**(1):27-38

[45] Vlychou M, Koutroumpas A, Malizos K, Sakkas LI. Ultrasonographic evidence of inflammation is frequent in hands of patients with erosive osteoarthritis. Osteoarthritis Cartilage. 2009;**17**(10):1283-1287

[46] Keen HI, Wakefield RJ, Conaghan PG. A systematic review of ultrasonography in osteoarthritis. Annals of the Rheumatic Diseases. 2009;**68**(5):611-619

[47] Iagnocco A, Filippucci E, Ossandon A, Ciapetti A, Salaffi F, Basili S, et al. High resolution ultrasonography in detection of bone erosions in patients with hand osteoarthritis. Journal of Rheumatology. 2005;**32**(12):2381-2383

[48] Möller I, Bong D, Naredo E, Filippucci E, Carrasco I, Moragues C, et al. Ultrasound in the study and monitoring of osteoarthritis. Osteoarthritis Cartilage. 2008;**16**:S4-S7

[49] Tanamas SK, Jones G. Imaging of knee osteoarthritis. Clinical Practice. 2010;7(6):635

[50] Oo WM, Bo MT. Role of ultrasonography in knee osteoarthritis. Journal of Clinical Rheumatology: Practical Reports on Rheumatic & Musculoskeletal Diseases. 2016;**22**(6):324-329

[51] Keen HI, Wakefield RJ, Grainger AJ, Hensor EMA, Emery P, Conaghan PG. Can ultrasonography improve on radiographic assessment in osteoarthritis of the hands? A comparison between radiographic and ultrasonographic detected pathology. Annals of the Rheumatic Diseases. 2008;**67**(8):1116-1120

[52] Manaster BJ. Soft tissue tumors of the musculoskeletal system. In: Oncologic Imaging. 2nd ed. London, UK: Elsevier Health Sciences; 2002. pp. 668-694

[53] Nieminen HJ, Salmi A, Karppinen P, Hæggström E, Hacking SA. The potential utility of high-intensity ultrasound to treat osteoarthritis. Osteoarthritis Cartilage. 2014;**22**(11):1784-1799

[54] Huang M-H, Lin Y-S, Lee C-L, Yang R-C. Use of ultrasound to increase effectiveness of isokinetic exercise for knee osteoarthritis. Archives of Physical Medicine and Rehabilitation. 2005;**86**(8):1545-1551

[55] Ulus Y, Tander B, Akyol Y, Durmus D, Buyukakıncak O, Gul U, et al. Therapeutic ultrasound versus sham ultrasound for the management of patients with knee osteoarthritis: A randomized double-blind controlled clinical study. International Journal of Rheumatic Diseases. 2012;**15**(2):197-206

[56] Tascioglu F, Kuzgun S, Armagan O, Ogutler G. Short-term effectiveness of ultrasound therapy in knee osteoarthritis. Journal of International Medical Research. 2010;**38**(4):1233-1242

[57] Di Sante L, Paoloni M, Dimaggio M, Colella L, Cerino A, Bernetti A, et al. Ultrasound-guided aspiration and corticosteroid injection compared to horizontal therapy for treatment of knee osteoarthritis complicated with Baker's cyst: A randomized, controlled trial. European Journal of Physical and Rehabilitation Medicine. 2012;**48**(4):561-567

[58] Kozanoglu E, Basaran S, Guzel R, Guler-Uysal F. Short term efficacy of ibuprofen phonophoresis versus continuous ultrasound therapy in knee

osteoarthritis. Swiss Medical Weekly. 2003;**133**(23-24):333-338

[59] Nieminen HJ, Salmi A, Rinta-Aho J, Hubbel G, Wjuga K, Suuronen J-P, et al. MHz ultrasonic drive-in: Localized drug delivery for osteoarthritis therapy. In: 2013 IEEE International Ultrasonics Symposium (IUS). 2013. pp. 619-622

[60] Faisal AI, Majumder S, Mondal T, Cowan D, Naseh S, Deen MJ. Monitoring methods of human body joints: State-of-the-art and research challenges. Sensors. 2019;**19**(11):2629

[61] Chu ML, Gradisar IA, Railey MR, Bowling GF. Detection of knee joint diseases using acoustical pattern recognition technique. Journal of Biomechanics. 1976;**9**(3):111-114

[62] Kraft D, Knaack F, Bader R, Portwich R, Eichstaedt P, Bieber G. A survey on vibration and sound analysis for disease detection of knee and hip joints. In: Proceedings of the 6th International Workshop on Sensor-based Activity Recognition and Interaction [Internet]. Rostock, Germany: Association for Computing Machinery (iWOAR '19). 2019. pp. 1-9. DOI: 10.1145/3361684.3361686

[63] Blodgett WE. Auscultation of the knee joint. Boston Medical and Surgical Journal. 1902;**146**(3):63-66

[64] Mollan RAB, Mccullagh GC, Wilson RI. A critical appraisal of auscultation of human joints. Clinical Orthopaedics. 1982;**170**:231-237

[65] Bassiouni HM. Phonoarthrography: A new technique for recording joint sounds. In: Osteoarthritis-Diagnosis, Treatment and Surgery. IntechOpen; 2012. Available from: https://www.intechopen.com/books/osteoarthritis-diagnosis-treatment-and-surgery/phonoarthrography-a-new-technique-for-recording-joint-sounds

[66] Abbott SC. The use of multi dimensional attribute analysis to account for intense variability in phono arthrometric traces [Internet] [PhD thesis]. Anglia Ruskin University; 2008. Available from: https://ethos.bl.uk/OrderDetails.do?uin=uk.bl.ethos.493141

[67] Bocking G. The use of phonoarthrometry to detect osteoarthritis in the human knee joint: A clinical proof of concept study [Internet] [doctoral]. Anglia Ruskin University; 2013. Available from: https://arro.anglia.ac.uk/701465/

[68] Reddy NP, Rothschild BM, Mandal M, Gupta V, Suryanarayanan S. Noninvasive acceleration measurements to characterize knee arthritis and chondromalacia. Annals of Biomedical Engineering. 1995;**23**(1):78-84

[69] Tavathia S, Rangayyan RM, Frank CB, Bell GD, Ladly KO, Zhang YT. Analysis of knee vibration signals using linear prediction. IEEE Transactions on Biomedical Engineering. 1992;**39**(9):959-970

[70] Silva J, Chau T. Coupled microphone-accelerometer sensor pair for dynamic noise reduction in MMG signal recording. Electronics Letters. 2003;**39**(21):1496-1498

[71] Andersen RE, Arendt-Nielsen L, Madeleine P. A review of engineering aspects of vibroarthography of the knee joint. Critical Reviews in Physical Rehabilitation Medicine. 2016;**28**(1-2):13-32. Available from: http://www.dl.begellhouse.com/journals/757fcb0219d89390,7d05545f5ad8aa9c,47e4a7bb4f6fe824.html

[72] Befrui N, Elsner J, Flesser A, Huvanandana J, Jarrousse O, Le TN, et al. Vibroarthrography for early detection of knee osteoarthritis using normalized frequency features. Medical & Biological Engineering & Computing. 2018;**56**(8):1499-1514

[73] Wu Y, Chen P, Luo X, Huang H, Liao L, Yao Y, et al. Quantification of knee vibroarthrographic signal irregularity associated with patellofemoral joint cartilage pathology based on entropy and envelope amplitude measures. Computer Methods and Programs in Biomedicine. 2016;**130**:1-12

[74] Klemm L, Sühn T, Spiller M, Illanes A, Boese A, Friebe M. Improved acquisition of vibroarthrographic signals of the knee joint. In: 2019 41st Annual International Conference of the IEEE Engineering in Medicine and Biology Society (EMBC). 2019. pp. 1259-1262

[75] McCoy GF, McCrea JD, Beverland DE, Kernohan WG, Mollan RA. Vibration arthrography as a diagnostic aid in diseases of the knee. A preliminary report. Journal of Bone and Joint Surgery. British. 1987;**69**(2):288-293

[76] Rangayyan RM, Wu YF. Screening of knee-joint vibroarthrographic signals using statistical parameters and radial basis functions. Medical & Biological Engineering & Computing. 2008;**46**(3):223-232

[77] Madeleine P, Andersen RE, Larsen JB, Arendt-Nielsen L, Samani A. Wireless multichannel vibroarthrographic recordings for the assessment of knee osteoarthritis during three activities of daily living. Clinical Biomechanics (Bristol, Avon). 2020;**72**:16-23

[78] Andersen RE, Arendt-Nielsen L, Madeleine P. Knee joint vibroarthrography of asymptomatic subjects during loaded flexion-extension movements. Medical & Biological Engineering & Computing. 2018;**56**(12):2301-2312

[79] Rangayyan RM. Biomedical Signal Analysis. 2nd ed. New York, USA: Wiley; 2015

[80] Zhang YT, Rangayyan RM, Frank CB, Bell GD. Adaptive cancellation of muscle contraction interference in vibroarthrographic signals. IEEE Transactions on Biomedical Engineering. 1994;**41**(2):181-191

[81] Kim KS, Seo JH, Kang JU, Song CG. An enhanced algorithm for knee joint sound classification using feature extraction based on time-frequency analysis. Computer Methods and Programs in Biomedicine. 2009;**94**(2):198-206

[82] Rangayyan RM, Wu Y. Screening of knee-joint vibroarthrographic signals using probability density functions estimated with Parzen windows. Biomedical Signal Processing and Control. 2010;**5**(1):53-58

[83] Krishnan S, Rangayyan RM, Bell GD, Frank CB. Adaptive time-frequency analysis of knee joint vibroarthrographic signals for noninvasive screening of articular cartilage pathology. IEEE Transactions on Biomedical Engineering. 2000;**47**(6):773-783

[84] Xie S, Krishnan S. Wavelet-based sparse functional linear model with applications to EEGs seizure detection and epilepsy diagnosis. Medical & Biological Engineering & Computing. 2013;**51**(1-2):49-60

[85] Krishnan S, Rangayyan RM, Bell GD, Frank CB, Ladly KO. Adaptive filtering, modelling and classification of knee joint vibroarthrographic signals for non-invasive diagnosis of articular cartilage pathology. Medical & Biological Engineering & Computing. 1997;**35**(6):677-684

[86] Nalband S, Sundar A, Prince AA, Agarwal A. Feature selection and classification methodology for the detection of knee-joint disorders. Computer Methods and Programs in Biomedicine. 2016;**127**:94-104

[87] Kręcisz K, Bączkowicz D. Analysis and multiclass classification of pathological knee joints using vibroarthrographic signals. Computer Methods and Programs in Biomedicine. 2018;**154**:37-44

[88] Karaduman D, Bircan DA, Çetin A. Assessment of crack initiation and propagation in bone using acoustic emission (AE) techniques. Journal of Mechanics in Medicine and Biology. 2018;**18**(03):1850031

[89] Aggelis DG, Paschos NK, Barkoula NM, Paipetis AS, Matikas TE, Georgoulis AD. Rupture of anterior cruciate ligament monitored by acoustic emission. Journal of the Acoustical Society of America. 2011;**129**(6):EL217-EL222

[90] Strantza M, Polyzos D, Louis O, Boulpaep F, Van Hemelrijck D, Aggelis DG. Damage characterization on human femur bone by means of ultrasonics and acoustic emission. Journal of Physics: Conference Proceedings. Ghent, Belgium. 2015

[91] Schwalbe HJ, Bamfaste G, Franke RP. Non-destructive and non-invasive observation of friction and wear of human joints and of fracture initiation by acoustic emission. Proceedings of the Institution of Mechanical Engineers. 1999;**213**(1):41-48

[92] Inan OT, Hersek S, Teague CN, Toreyin H, Jeong HK, Jones ML, et al. A stethoscope for the knee: Investigating joint acoustical emissions as novel biomarkers for wearable joint health assessment. Journal of the Acoustical Society of America. 2016;**139**(4):2175-2176

[93] Choi D, Ahn S, Ryu J, Nagao M, Kim Y. Knee acoustic emission characteristics of the healthy and the patients with osteoarthritis using piezoelectric sensor. Sensors and Materials. 2018;**30**(8):1629-1641

[94] Töreyin H, Jeong HK, Hersek S, Teague CN, Inan OT. Quantifying the consistency of wearable knee acoustical emission measurements during complex motions. IEEE Journal of Biomedical and Health Informatics. 2016;**20**(5):1265-1272

[95] Töreyin H, Hersek S, Teague CN, Inan OT. A proof-of-concept system to analyze joint sounds in real time for knee health assessment in uncontrolled settings. IEEE Sensors Journal. 2016;**16**(9):2892-2893

[96] Teague CN, Hersek S, Toreyin H, Millard-Stafford ML, Jones ML, Kogler GF, et al. Novel methods for sensing acoustical emissions from the knee for wearable joint health assessment. IEEE Transactions on Biomedical Engineering. 2016;**63**(8):1581-1590

[97] Jeong HK, Whittingslow D, Inan OT. b-Value: A potential biomarker for assessing knee-joint health using acoustical emission sensing. IEEE Sensors Letters. 2018;**2**(4):1-4

[98] Feng G-H, Chen W-M. Piezoelectric-film-based acoustic emission sensor array with thermoactuator for monitoring knee joint conditions. Sensors and Actuators A: Physical. 2016;**246**:180-191

[99] Mascaro B, Prior J, Shark L-K, Selfe J, Cole P, Goodacre J. Exploratory study of a non-invasive method based on acoustic emission for assessing the dynamic integrity of knee joints. Medical Engineering & Physics. 2009;**31**(8):1013-1022

[100] Schlüter DK, Spain L, Quan W, Southworth H, Platt N, Mercer J, et al. Use of acoustic emission to identify novel candidate biomarkers for knee osteoarthritis (OA). PLoS One.

2019;**14**(10):e0223711. Available from: https://www.ncbi.nlm.nih.gov/pmc/articles/PMC6795455/

[101] Bączkowicz D, Skiba G, Szmajda M, Vařeka I, Falkowski K, Laudner K. Effects of viscosupplementation on quality of knee joint arthrokinematic motion analyzed by vibroarthrography. Cartilage. 2019;**9**:1947603519847737

[102] Karpiński R, Machrowska A, Maciejewski M. Application of acoustic signal processing methods in detecting differences between open and closed kinematic chain movement for the knee joint. Applied Computer Science. 2019;**15**(1):36-48. Available from: http://yadda.icm.edu.pl/baztech/element/bwmeta1.element.baztech-2a2ddb8c-96f9-4f3e-97a4-a73196b5971d

[103] Shark L-K, Chen H, Goodacre J. Discovering differences in acoustic emission between healthy and osteoarthritic knees using a four-phase model of sit-stand-sit movements. Open Medical Informatics Journal. 2010;**4**:116-125

[104] Wiens AD, Prahalad S, Inan OT. Vibro CV: A computer vision-based vibroarthrography platform with possible application to juvenile idiopathic arthritis. In: Conference Proceedings: Annual International Conference of the IEEE Engineering in Medicine and Biology Society. IEEE Engineering in Medicine and Biology Society; 2016. 2016. pp. 4431-4434

[105] Goodacre J, Schlueter D, Shark L-K, Spain L, Platt N, Platt N, et al. 097 Identifying novel acoustic emission biomarkers for use in knee osteoarthritis clinical trials. Rheumatology. 2018;**57**(suppl_3):key075-321. Available from: insights.ovid.com

[106] Adouni M, Shirazi-Adl A. Knee joint biomechanics in closed-kinetic-chain exercises. Computer Methods in Biomechanics and Biomedical Engineering. 2009;**12**(6):661-670

Chapter 4

Control of a Prosthetic Arm Using fNIRS, a Neural-Machine Interface

Usama Ali Syed, Zareena Kausar and Neelum Yousaf Sattar

Abstract

Development in the field of bio-mechatronics has provided diverse ways to mimic and improve the function of human limbs. Without an elbow joint, the hand remains stiff because all the muscles tension passes through this joint. Advanced myoelectric prosthetic devices are limited due to the lack of appropriate signal sources on residual amputee muscles and insufficient real-time control. Neural-machine interfaces (NMI) are representing a recent approach to develop effective applications. In this research study, an NMI is designed that presents real-time signal processing for command generation. The human brain hemodynamic responses are, therefore, translated into control commands for people suffering from trans-humeral amputation. A novel and first of its kind scheme is proposed which utilizes functional near-infrared spectroscopy (fNIRS) to generate the control commands for a three-degree-of-freedom (DOF) prosthetic arm. The time window for fNIRS signals was set to 1 second. The average accuracy was found to be 82% which is a state-of-the-art result for such a technique. The accuracy ranged from 65 to 85% subject-wise. The data were trained and tested on both artificial neural network (ANN) and linear discriminant analysis (LDA). Eight out of 10 motions were correctly predicted in real time by both classifiers.

Keywords: functional near-infrared spectroscopy (fNIRS), real-time signal processing, upper-limb prosthesis, transhumeral amputees, artificial neural network, linear discriminant analysis

1. Introduction

Amputation is taken from the Latin terminology "amputare" meaning to cut out. It is a removal of a limb due to medical reasons such as diseases and accidents. After this, an artificial device (prosthetics) is provided to fulfill all the desired needs. A prosthesis is an artificial device that replaces a missing body part that may be lost due to any traumatic accidents or medical reasons.

In the nineteenth century, hooks and wooden limbs were used as a replacement to fulfill the supporting needs to overcome support as well as the psychological effects experienced during the time. Prosthetic arm is a biomedical device consisting of links and joints in an open or closed system, which is also a combination of electronics. Thus, there is a need for a specified prosthetic which would help in fulfilling the requirements of the patient.

Types of amputation	Types of prosthesis
Shoulder disarticulation	From shoulder below the elbow
Transhumeral	Above elbow
Transradial	Below elbow
Transcarpal	Below elbow

Table 1.
Types of upper-limb amputation and respective prosthesis type.

Prosthetics also come under different categories concerning the patient's demand and desirable need. **Table 1** lists the type of amputation and their respective prosthesis type.

Controlling a prosthetic arm could be done in several ways. Some of them are by using Invasive Methods, which reflects a process in which an instrument is introduced in the human body. In such a process, electrodes are implanted inside the body, which would receive and implement the process. The other referred to as the non-invasive method. A non-invasion process does not introduce instruments into the body but uses the surface information to get its details and the desired output that is to be determined.

In the previous studies, various strategies have been practiced to monitor muscle activations all through activities, as reported by Lobo Prat et al. [1] To carry out a valuation of muscular contraction, sonomyography (SMG), mechanomyography (MMG) [2, 3], miokinemetric (MK), and electric impedance estimations are classically applied. Though muscular intentions and/or contraction are often determined using electromyography (EMG) and near-infrared spectroscopy (NIRS) [4], it allows continuous monitoring of the muscle during motor actions or rehabilitative movements. Further practices, such as ultrasonography [5] and lactate sampling, offer only a representation of the muscular status at the moment of the study, and not an effective trace in time.

Optical brain imaging is a frequently applied methodology in human-machine interaction technically acknowledged as functional near-infrared spectroscopy (fNIRS). It allows them to monitor the quantification of the relative changes in concentration of oxygenated and deoxygenated hemoglobin in tissue blood based on artificial diffuse spectroscopy. Functional neuroimaging suggests a non-invasive method of indirect as well as direct monitoring of brain activity. The hardware involved is portable hence making it easy to carry out experiments in any environment. fNIRS is a non-invasive brain imaging method including the quantification of chromophore concentration determined from the measurement of near-infrared (NIR) light attenuation or time-based changes [6]. It exploits the optical window in which the fundamental elements found in the human body typically cause no hindrance to infrared light of small wavelength range that is 700–900 nm. In addition to that, oxygenated hemoglobin (Hb) and deoxygenated-hemoglobin (deoxy-Hb) are strong absorbers of light which are the key components to translate the brain response [7]. The peculiarity in the absorption bands of deoxy-Hb and oxy-Hb permit the estimation of near changes in hemoglobin concentration by methods of estimating light attenuation at a couple of known wavelengths [8]. The reason behind choosing more than one wavelength is to take care of the isosbestic point that occurs at around 810 nm. At this value of light wavelength both the absorbing coefficients are indistinguishable [9].

Via the improved Beer-Lambert law [10], relative concentration is evaluated concerning the entire length covered by the light photon [11, 12]. Now, for an

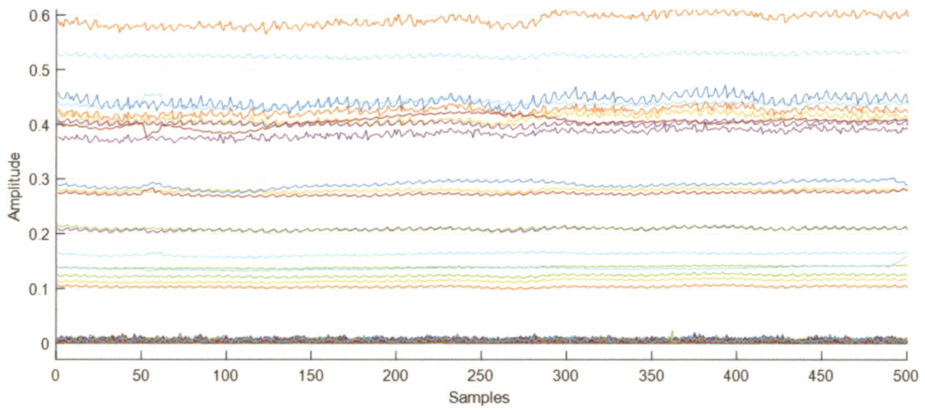

Figure 1.
Raw fNIRS light intensity.

incident ray of light an emitter and to detect that reflected light, a detector is positioned. The distance between them is also defined. Hence, a state of brain hemodynamic is captured. The raw light concentrations that are further transformed into hemodynamic responses by the implementation of renowned Beer-Lambert Law and further utilized for feature extraction and classification. The extracted light intensity patterns can be viewed in **Figure 1**.

Several research institutions have undertaken the design and construction of robotic arms. These structures diverge depending upon the proposed utilization of the human hand. Diverse knowledge of actuation approaches has been considered and implemented. Earlier design approaches have focused on the mechanical problems of the construction and operation of the prosthetic devices. Most of these hardware devices are controlled via methods that are not natural, such as using the contraction of muscles of the opposite arm. This research attempts to lay the foundation for a scheme that can offer functionality similar to the human arm, with an intuitive technique of control.

A search carried out using Web of Science engine, to review work done in this area along with the gap identification, revealed no work done so far in this field of study.

2. Materials and methods

The human arm is capable of performing seven basic motions associated with joints in the human arm. To account for transhumeral amputation, three of the main arm motions are considered i.e. one elbow and two motions affiliated with the wrist joint. These motions comprise wrist extension (WE), elbow flexion (EF), wrist supination (WS), wrist flexion (WF), elbow extension (EE), and wrist pronation (WP).

This section elaborates on the data acquisition of the defined motions. These motions were captured using The NIRsport manufactured by NIRx Technologies. It is an accessible, segmental, and robust functional near-infrared spectroscopy (fNIRS) machine that measures hemodynamic responses generated by neuro-activation of the inside brain via oxy-, deoxy-, and total hemoglobin variations in the cerebral cortex.

The updated version, NIRsport-2 proposes a host prepared to implement advancements and units to meet the requirements of wide-ranging cognitive neuroscience applications. The major advantage of this device is that it is designed to work in a rugged environment and also this device is portable. This feature aids in the development of a wearable and portable system.

2.1 Sample

A total of 15 healthy subjects were engaged who were reported to be right-hand dominant males having a mean age of 30 with a standard deviation of 4. Righthanders had been pursued to confine any dissimilarities in the hemodynamic responses because of the hemispheric domination difference [13]. All participants were chosen wisely as no one of the selected subjects had engaged in any prior study associated with brain signal acquisition experiments. None was accounted for to have a past filled with any mental, neurological, or visual affliction. Every one of them had an ordinary vision, and all signed and agreed to a composed consent after being briefed in detail regarding the test procedure. Three amputee subjects also participated in the study. Their demographics are given in **Table 2**.

Trials employing fNIRS were permitted by the Air University Human Research Ethics Committee (HREC). These research experiments were held regarding ethical standards dictated by the world medical association in the recent declaration of Helsinki [14].

The generic methodology can be seen in **Figure 2**.

2.2 fNIRS data acquisition

2.2.1 Preparation

The specially designed fNIRS headset i.e. Easycap by NIRx technologies follows the international standard of source-detector separations i.e. 3 cm [15–24]. After the subject wears the cap, the optodes are calibrated. The result of this calibration can be analyzed as in **Figure 3**. The faulty setting is shown in **Figure 3(b)**. The boxes represent optodes. The color bar indicates if the optodes are in contact with the scalp or not and hence the colors are assigned. The white color depicts no connection between scalp and optodes. The red color indicated that the connection between the scalp and optode is critical, i.e. it needs to be adjusted. Sometimes hair comes as a hindrance and just by plugging the optode again in the cap would help establish a better connection. If the issue is not resolved by then, a clinical gel (EASYCAP Supervisc, high-viscosity electrolyte-gel) is used to make sure no hair absorbed the light. The gel is rated healthy and is safe to use with optodes. The yellow color indicates that the connection is acceptable. The signals can be acquired. In this scenario, the machine conditions are calibrated by the machine itself. The machine adds a gain factor to the optodes where the connection is acceptable and it

Patient ID	A1	A2	A3
Gender	Male	Male	Male
Age	23	32	42
Amputated side	Right	Left	Right
Residual length (cm)	14	18	10
Time of amputation (months)	7	24	145

Table 2.
Demographic characteristics of amputed subjects.

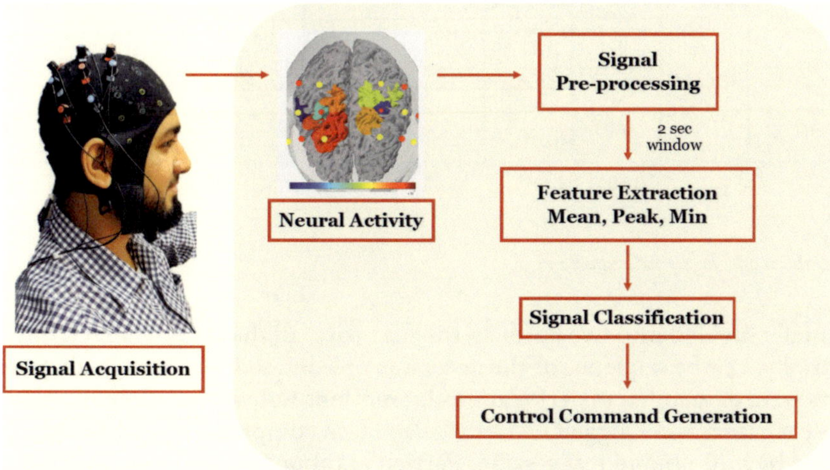

Figure 2.
Generic methodology.

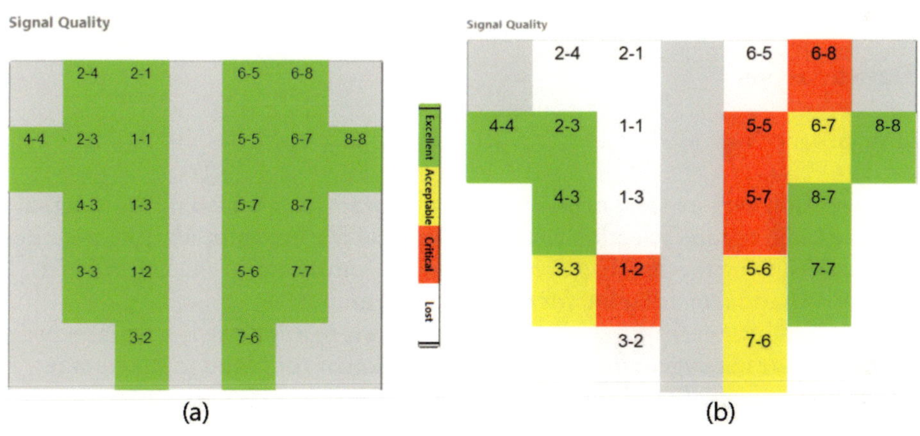

Figure 3.
Visual representation of optode settings. The perfect setting is illustrated in (a) meanwhile the faulty optode settings are shown in (b). The color bar on the right side represents the signal quality class.

is saved in conditions file which is used in signal processing later. The green color shows that the optodes are perfectly placed on the head surface and an excellent connection is established for data acquisition. It can be analyzed in **Figure 3(a)**.

2.2.2 Acquisition

When the optodes are aligned, signal acquisition is started. The test strategy was segmented into training and testing. The subjects were asked to complete six tasks that were identified by fNIRS.

A comfortable chair was set up roughly 100 cm away from the subjects so that the motion cues are visible to them while the screen backlight does not interfere with the optical sensors [25–38]. This environment was set up for signal extraction. The Easycap was prepared in advance to minimize the time consumption during the optode placement process. Yet some of the detectors/sources had to be optimized during the calibration process by fixing hair via gel. The session commenced with an undeveloped span of 30 seconds to create a reference point. Later the screen indicated the participants to perform one of six definite tasks the training was

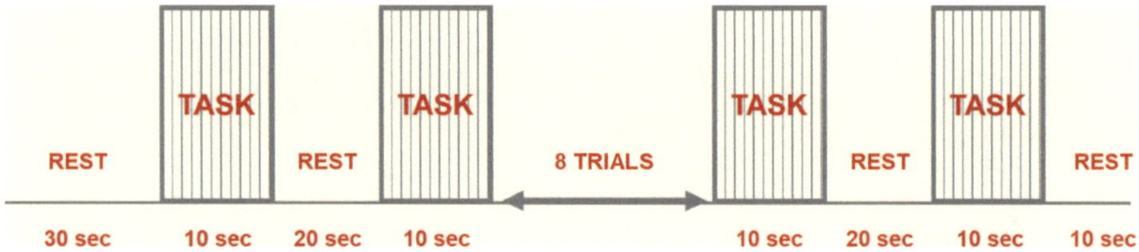

Figure 4.
Experimental model for signal acquisition.

additionally divided into two parts. In the first part, all the tasks were recorded sequentially, i.e. the sequence of the tasks was pre-defined. In the second stage, the subjects were demanded to perform similar motions but with random intentions. All these six tasks were logged by fNIRS. Each task comprised of 10-second trials separated by a 20-second rest session. Particulars about the experimental model are given below in **Figure 4**.

The acquired data was then processed and is briefly illustrated in the coming section.

3. Data analysis

3.1 Pre-processing

This section explores and explains the signal processing which includes signal pre-processing, optode selection criteria, statistical feature computation, and the signal classification method to generate a control command for the control of a 3-DOF prosthetic arm designed for transhumeral amputees.

Functional near-infrared spectroscopy is the raw light intensity values recorded during a change in oxygenation and de-oxygenation of the blood in the human brain. With the help of dual-tip optodes, this concentration is recorded with two different wavelengths i.e. 760 and 850 nm. In the nirsLAB environment, the data is further processed. nirsLAB is the signal processing software that comes with the machine. nirsLAB is fully aware of the specifications and conditions applied during signal acquisition, hence the best choice for signal processing. The unwanted data is truncated along with unusual spikes or discontinuities that occurred during acquisition. It is then filtered to compute the hemodynamic states. These hemodynamic states are now utilized to extract the features.

As soon as the light intensities are acquired, they are fed to nirsLAB where first the time of stimulus is defined which in our case is 10 seconds as per the designed experimental paradigm. The data is further marked according to the conditions i.e. motion and rest.

Figure 5 represents the raw fNIRS data of both wavelengths i.e. 760 and 850 nm. It is evident that the amplitude for both data sets is different as the concentration of hemodynamic response is varying from healthy to the amputated subject. This is because of the absence of an arm. As the brain generates these signals, the unwanted responses die due to the absence of neuron carrier in the brain. The connection of arm and brain is cut because there is nothing present at the receiving end. Further, the discontinuities are removed along with the spikes if there exists any. The data is then fed for filtration. nirsLAB provides the commonly practiced filters for fNIRS data. Band-pass filter was implemented to smooth the acquired light intensities. The filtered and raw data at both the wavelengths are illustrated below in **Figure 6**.

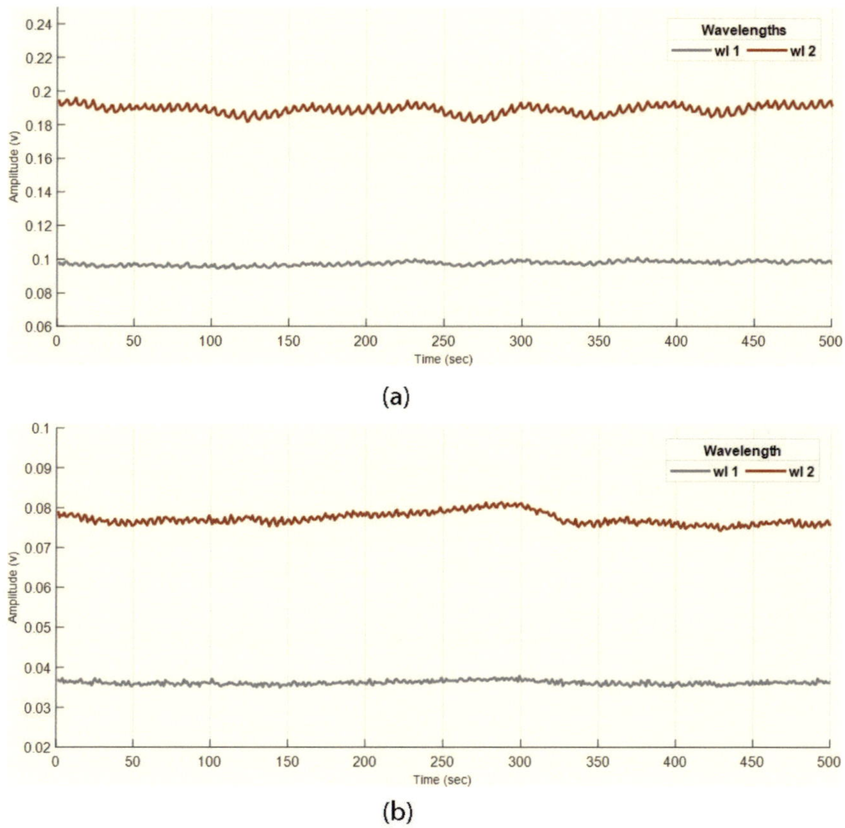

Figure 5.
The first chunk of fNIRS data according to the defined experimental paradigm is illustrated. The initial and final rest is truncated. (a) fNIRS signals of healthy subjects and (b) fNIRS signals acquired from amputee subject.

nirsLAB makes use of firls and filtfilt MATLAB® commands to filter the data. firls returns the parameters of a linear-phase filter, while filtfilt applies the filter parameters into the data. The latter is set to work as finite impulse response (FIR). The roll-off defines the width of the transition frequency band, i.e. how steep the transition between frequencies which are cut and frequencies which are passed for each of the upper and lower limits of frequency. The width of the transition band is calculated as Eqs. (1) and (2):

$$\text{Upper limit} = 1 + \frac{Roll-off}{2} \quad (1)$$

$$\text{Lower limit} = 1 - \frac{Roll-off}{2} \quad (2)$$

This noise-free and minimum artifact data are then used to find the hemodynamic states by using the modified Beer-Lambert Law [10, 39–41].

This light intensity raw data is then used to compute the hemodynamic response of the brain. The hemodynamic changes computed offline in nirsLAB are based on the modified Beer-Lambert law for scattering media, as mentioned above. While in nirsLAB the operator can modify all input parameters of the Beer-Lambert law

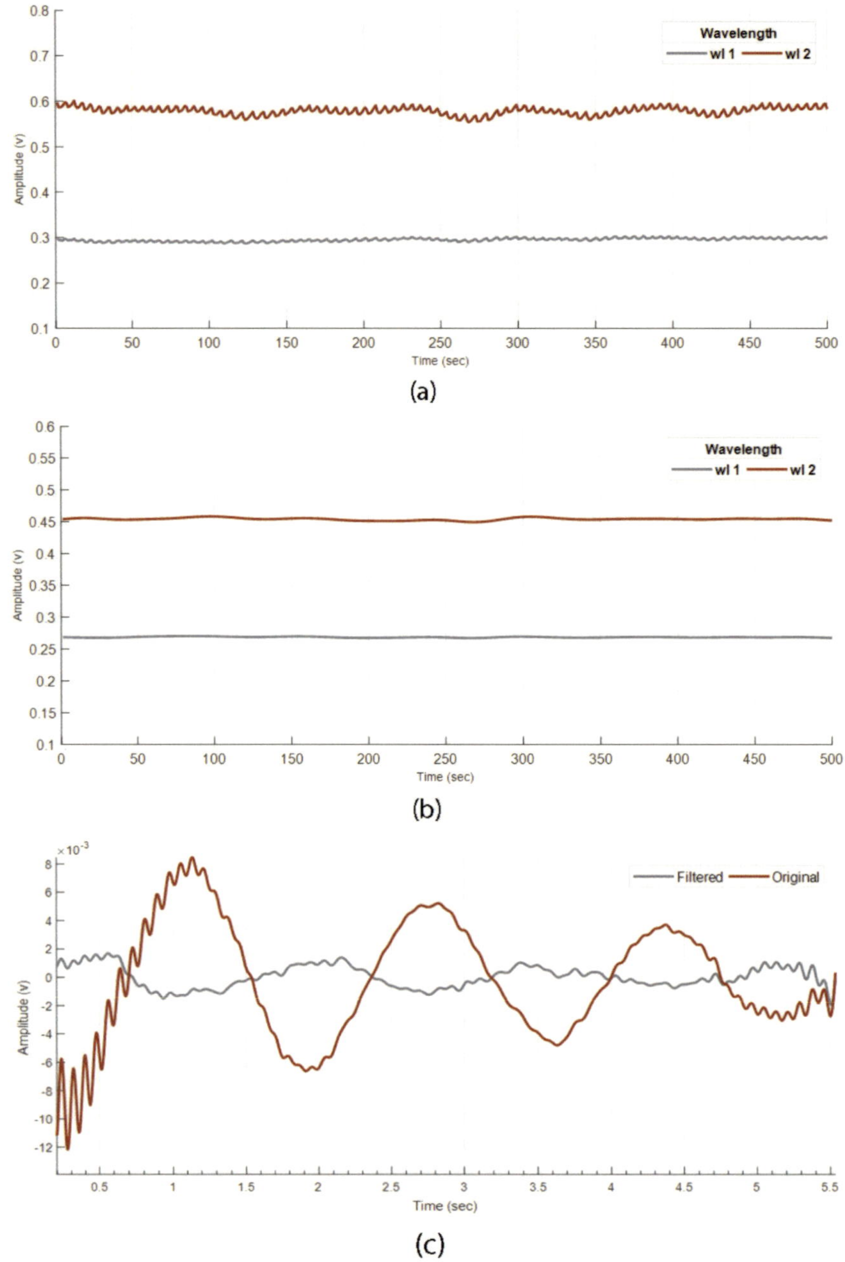

Figure 6.
(a) The filtered data for both wavelengths after filtering can be seen in this illustration. Band-pass filter has range of 0.01–0.2 Hz. The roll-off was set to 15 as a default value. (b) The same signal is smoothed and as it is a large time-series, (c) a chunk of signal for a closer look is illustrated which is for the first 5 seconds of the activity during the task.

(absorption coefficients and inter-optode distance), in NIRStar®, these are fixed, as they are calculated real-time. More precisely, the values for real-time ΔHbO and ΔHb computation are as follows:

Absorption coefficients are 3.843707 and 1.4865865 for 760 nm, deoxy and oxy, respectively, and for 850 nm, 1.798643 and 2.526391 deoxy and oxy, respectively.

The default inter-optode distance is set to 3.0 cm and the absorption coefficient unit is millimole per liter per centimeter (1/cm)/(mmol/L).

Mathematically, it is defined as Eq. (3)

$$\Delta A(\lambda) = \varepsilon(\lambda).\Delta c.d.DPF(\lambda) + g(\lambda) \tag{3}$$

where the variables can be defined as A: light reduction, or $\Delta A(\lambda)$: changes in light reduction at a given wavelength (λ); $\varepsilon(\lambda)$: loss of the chromophore at a certain wavelength (λ); Δc: changes observed in the chromophore absorption; d: distance between source and detector; $DPF(\lambda)$: differential path length factor (DPF) for a certain wavelength (λ); $g(\lambda)$: the scattering of the light wave at a certain wavelength (λ), where g is annulled since it is presumed to be insignificant when only light attenuation (as in continuous-wave NIRS) is considered [20, 36, 42–47].

The differential path length factor (DPF) is a dimensionless modification factor that takes care of the increase in the optical path length that is produced by the scattering of light in organic tissue. The product of DPF and source-detector separation evaluates the "true" path length that the light has traveled inside the biological tissue cell [37, 38, 48, 49]. For NIRx technologies, this value is set constant for wavelengths 7.25/6.38 for 760/850 nm respectively.

3.2 Feature extraction

The mathematical representation of statistical features extracted during the study is given as follows.

Signal mean (SM) was computed as Eq. (4)

$$SM = \frac{1}{N}\sum_{i=1}^{N} X_i \tag{4}$$

where N denotes the length of the data points within a segment and X_i represents the signal values.

Signal peak (SP) is defined by the change in signals amplitude among two adjacent segments which surpass a predefined threshold to reduce noise. It is given by Eq. (5)

$$SP = \sum_{i=1}^{N} f\left(\left|X_i - X_{i+1}\right|\right) \tag{5}$$

where N represents the samples while X_i and X_{i+1} represent the successive peaks in the signal. These features are extracted and fed to the classifier to predict the motion.

4. Classification process

The statistical features extracted from the data sample are then fed to the classifier. Classifying methods are employed to predict the motion intention. To comprehensively evaluate the performance of features, the two widely used classifiers in pattern recognition were implemented, namely, linear discriminant analysis (LDA) and artificial neural network (ANN). A generic yet comprehensive process is illustrated in **Figure 7**.

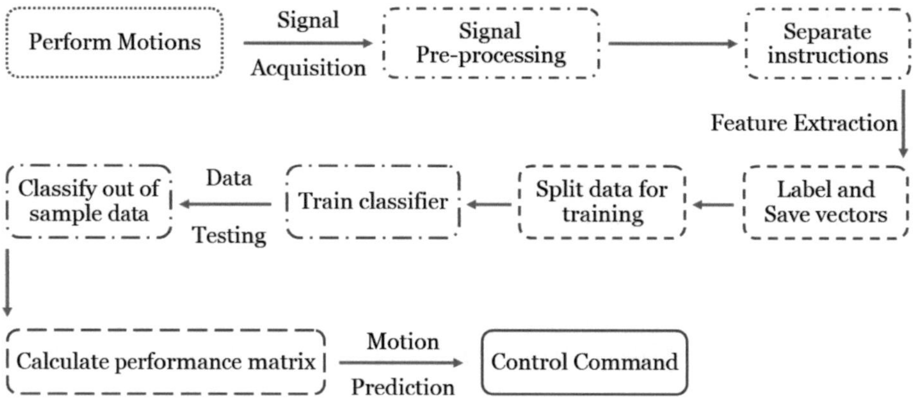

Figure 7.
A generic classification process.

4.1 Linear discriminant analysis

Fisher's discriminant analysis or linear discriminant analysis is a method used to dimensionally contract samples of two or more classes to separate them, linearly. This classification method projects all the samples on an imaginary line which is useful for data classification. To cater for the word linear, it suggests that the classifier will dimension the given samples to represent the class information. It characterizes the resulting combinations to reduce the number of arbitrary samples by tracing a set of values in a distinct form. It anticipates the sample information so that each class is isolated without any problem. It decreases intraclass variance and increases the interclass mean. By doing this, unlike data samples become segmented from each other and their set point shrinks together so that they cannot be mixed with other classes.

LDA is commonly used for pattern classification in offline and online systems. This technique projects all the data points on a line in such a way that each data sample that corresponds to a class is separated effectively. It decreases the intra-class variance and increases the inter-class mean. By doing this, different classes become separated from each other, and their data points get closer together so that they cannot be mixed with other classes. LDA works by maximizing the Fisher's criterion given in Eq. (6)

$$J(v) = \frac{v^t S_B\, v}{v^t S_w v} \tag{6}$$

Between classes scatter matrix S_B is defined as in Eq. (7)

$$S_B = \sum_{x_i}^{c} n_i (\mu_i - \mu)(\mu_i - \mu)^t \tag{7}$$

where n_i represents several samples that belong to class i, the class scatter matrix S_w is defined as in Eq. (8)

$$S_w = \sum_{x_i}^{c} S_i = \sum_{x_i}^{c} \sum_{x_k \in Class(i)} (x_k - \mu_i)(x_k - \mu_i)^t \tag{8}$$

A generalized eigenvector problem can be represented as Eq. (9)

$$S_B v = \lambda S_w v \tag{9}$$

The optimal v is the eigenvector corresponding to the largest eigenvalue can be written represented as in Eq. (10) provided that S_w is nonsingular.

$$v = S_W^{-1}(\mu_i - \mu) \tag{10}$$

The classifier results were validated using the cross-validation scheme. The number of folds/layers was set to 10. It means that the entire data was mixed randomly into 10 groups, out of which nine took part to train the classifier while one remains untouched for testing purposes. This process was repeated 10 times until all groups were tested against each other.

As an initial measure, the attributes of the dataset which need to be classified or dimensionally contracted will lead to the choice of applying this method as a classifier or a dimensionality reduction algorithm to play out any desired task. The primary thought of Fisher's analysis is fundamentally to isolate sample classes linearly moving them to an alternate feature-space. In this way, if the considered data set is linearly distinguishable, just using the algorithm as a classifier will yield better results. In any case, if the dataset is not truly distinct the classifier will attempt to sort out this dataset in another space. Yet despite every measure, the classes sample data may overlap due to the non-linear characteristic present in the sampled dataset. For this situation, there emerges a need to utilize another grouping model to manage nonlinearities governing the dataset. Hence, a neural network that comprise of hidden layers is also implemented. As for the neural network, raw data is used as input rather than featured data. This will give a broader idea of how to predict any output based on the input that have non-linear characteristic.

4.2 Artificial neural network (ANN)

ANN utilizes multiple neuron layers to map data from one distribution to another for better and optimized classification. A technique called backpropagation helps ANN to learn the relationship between input and output class label. The neural network toolbox provided by MATLAB® was utilized to train the classifier. First, network topology and an activation function were defined and then weights were randomized. The model uses all training data to approximate the error of the predicted output as compared to the actual output. Then it uses the error to adjust the weights so that it could be minimized for the next training data and this process was repeated until the error was minimized. For this network we employed Relu as the activation function; the weights were initialized using the Xavier distribution, the network utilized the Adam optimizer function for gradient descent. We used 60% of data for training, and 20% for testing and validation each. A confusion matrix was generated afterward, which had a class number corresponding to each arm motion. The number of hidden layers was specified i.e. 10, and system training was initiated. Ten neurons were present in each of the intermediate hidden layer. The number of neurons in output or last layer was set to be 6, which is equal to the number of elements in the target vector.

After classifying the information, their real-time testing was performed to ensure the behavior of both classifying techniques. But bear in mind that both of these classifiers have different parameters and methodologies. They are not compared with each other here but they are implemented to grasp a comprehensive idea of how these different brain hemodynamic intentions can be evaluated. LDA and ANN were both applied separately and the outcomes are discussed in next section.

5. Results and discussions

In research, the neural-machine interfaces can have a control foundation of either a single modality or via hybrid activity. This present study dwells on capturing hemodynamic responses from the human brain and generating the control command that can be translated to activate a prosthetic arm for transhumeral amputees. The results found by this particular research are discussed as follows.

These hemodynamic states are mapped using nirsLAB in **Figure 8**. The color bar represents the concentration of oxygenation.

5.1 Channel selection

The changes in oxygenated hemoglobin ΔHbO for all 20 channels and six activities of subject 6 are demonstrated in **Figure 9**. All of the optodes were not capturing the true concentration changes while brain activity was performed by the subject. Nevertheless, it was observed that similar channels were active when identical motions were executed while signal acquisition.

The channel outputs in **Figure 8** serve to highlight the need for choosing good channels for recognizing true brain activities. According to our channel choice standard, signal averaging was used. It is understandable by human brain studies that when the right side of the human body is in motion, the left hemisphere of

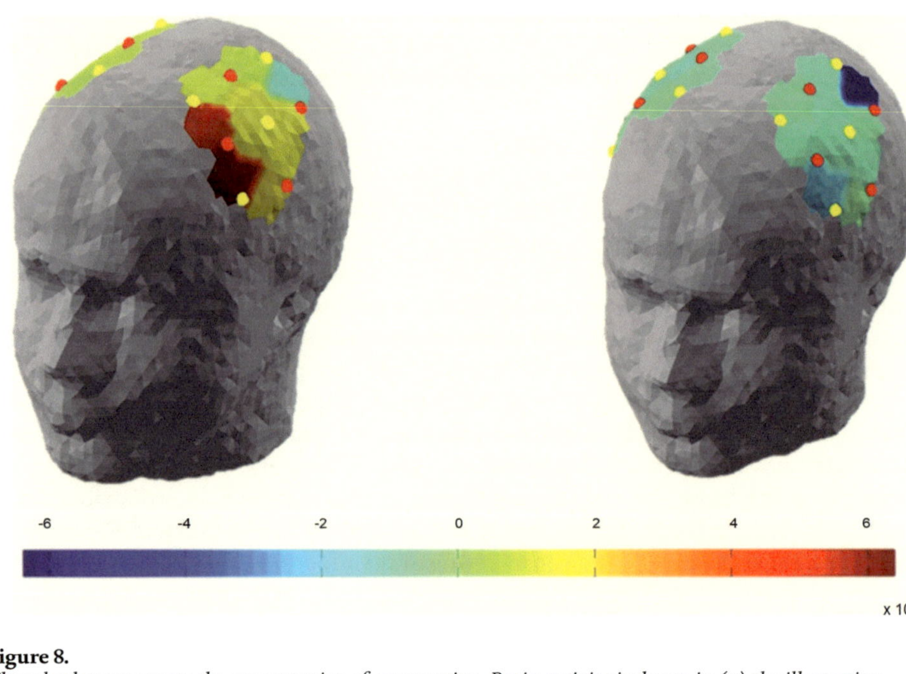

Figure 8.
The color bar represents the concentration of oxygenation. Brain activity is shown in (a) the illustration represents condition 1 i.e. motion. It can be seen that the motor region is "hot" when compared to the color bar. It depicts motion state whereas the (b) shows that the brain is undergoing significantly low or minimal hemodynamic changes hence the "cool" values depicting the condition 2 i.e. rest. The red and yellow dots seen in the motor cortex region are representations of optodes and they were positioned according to the international system.

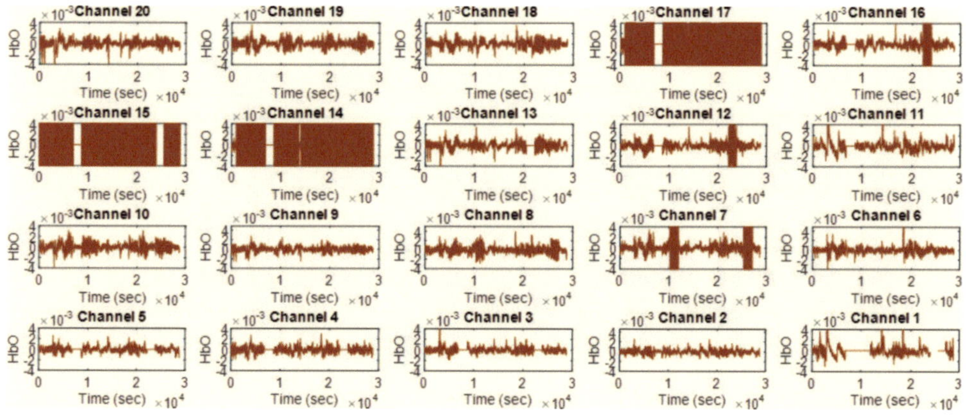

Figure 9.
Optode-wise hemodynamic status visualization.

the human brain is activated. As in our case, the subjects were asked to move their right hand, it is obvious that the hemodynamic patterns occurring in the right hemisphere are merely noise. It can be seen in **Figure 8** that all the channels of right hemisphere i.e. channels 1–10 do not show significant activity and later they were discarded while classification. The left side of the motor cortex was however active and the channels from 11 to 20 were used to extract the statistical features which took part in the classification. Features were computed spatially which allowed the overall brain activity on the left side of the motor cortex region of the human brain.

Window sizing of diverse spans has been utilized in several studies for the detection of fNIRS features [50, 51]. It is intended to minimize the window size to generate a fast response for real-time applications. So, the time spans of 0–0.5, 0–1, and 0–2 second windows were selected. These split seconds were employed for investigation of hemodynamic features to secure the best window size that will aid in decreased calculation time.

5.2 Classification accuracy

The stated performance outcomes were statistically evaluated based on the number of correctly predicted samples while the activity was completed during the period of 0–10 seconds. These actions were assessed by MATLAB® implementing the 10-fold cross-validation course. Student's t-test was performed to establish the statistical significance of the obtained results. The confidence interval was set to 95% ($p < 0.05$). The quantitative comparison between healthy subjects and amputees was not possible due to a limited number of amputees. The computed p-value was 0.0337 considering a 95% confidence interval. The classification accuracies of the subjects are shown in **Figure 10**.

A confusion matrix is illustrated in **Table 3** where it is evident that the wrist pronation and supination cause the most confusion. From time to time the subject executes the actions and sometimes put a break to them. In so doing the muscle intention power descend below the threshold and is not detected, and subsequently tagged as uncounted or undetected.

In common practices, in addition to muscular fatigue, mental fatigue could likewise show up. This would affect the unwavering quality of the fNIRS signal. Frequent use of nicotine substances involving tea or coffee and weak eyesight are

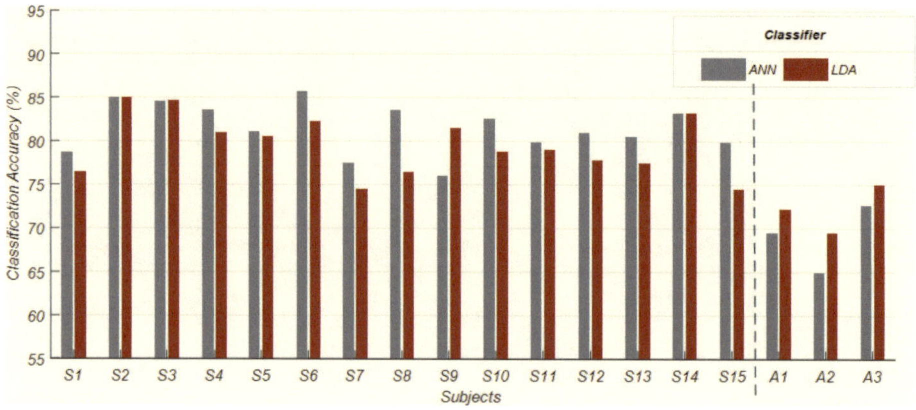

Figure 10.
A representation of subject-wise accuracies. Healthy subjects are presented as S1–S15 whereas amputees are labeled A1–A3. All concerning classifying technique as LDA and ANN.

Output class Target class	1	2	3	4	5	6
1	**5010** **100.0%**	0 0.0%	0 0.0%	0 0.0%	0 0.0%	0 0.0%
2	0 0.0%	**4978** **99.3%**	12 0.3%	0 0.0%	0 0.0%	0 0.0%
3	0 0.0%	0 0.0%	**3648** **73%**	720 14.4%	0 0.0%	0 0.0%
4	0 0.0%	20 0.4%	630 12.6%	**3617** **72.1%**	0 0.0%	0 0.0%
5	0 0.0%	0 0.0%	0 0.0%	0 0.0%	**5001** **99.8%**	0 0.0%
6	0 0.0%	0 0.0%	0 0.0%	23 0.5%	9 0.2%	**4978** **99.3%**

Table 3.
Confusion matrix of motion prediction.

accounted for in such reliability. The motion prediction accuracy of an individual can be changed under the influence of such conditions.

5.3 Control command generation

After the results from the classifier are returned, they are translated into a control command. The motions are assigned abbreviations identical as used in Section 2. They are listed here as in **Table 4**.

While testing, the machine responds as the variables illustrated in **Table 4** that are assigned to each class motion. The controllers further single-out one definitive motion which can be analyzed while testing the data.

These control commands can be further translated to motor action via a controller such as Arduino, Raspberry Pi, Odroid, etc. as the program routine is written in a language supported by all these controllers. A three degree of freedom device can be actuated using this neural-machine interface scheme.

To eliminate the channel selection part, manufacturers are working on bundled optodes. Using these bundled optodes will not only eliminate the channel selection

Motion	Notation
Extension of elbow	EE
Flexion of elbow	EF
Pronation of wrist	WP
Supination of wrist	WS
Flexion of wrist	WF

Table 4.
Class labels.

complications but it will also help in physical attributes as the whole head will not be covered. It will be easy to wear the head cap because of a smaller number of optodes and wires going around.

Also, using a different feature set may aid in the increase in accuracy. Rather than extracting three or four features, only one optimal feature can be evaluated. Hybridization of bio-signals can be done using advanced probability models or neural networks can be trained and implemented to hybridize different modalities.

6. Conclusion

fNIRS signals were acquired using the NIRSport machine developed by NIRx technology. These signals were recorded for six motions i.e. elbow extension (EE), elbow flexion (EF), wrist supination (WS), wrist pronation (WP), wrist extension (WE) and wrist flexion (WF) and were further analyzed. Mean and peak feature was extracted from the hemodynamic response of the brain. Also, minimum values were extracted for channel selection. The hemodynamic responses acquired from the brain were trained and tested by two widely used classifiers in pattern recognition i.e. LDA and ANN. The highest value of accuracy for an individual subject was recorded at 85% which is not yet achieved with six control commands employed by fNIRS. Both the classifiers were also active for real-time analysis. As a result of such high value of training accuracy, 8 out of 10 motions were correctly predicted in real-time setting. Possible extension of this work could be to hybridize these fNIRS signals together with another signal modality to not only increase the accuracy but also the number of control commands. Arm movement pattern for different age groups can be further explored. The number of amputed subjects could be increased to acquire data which will aid in better understanding of hemodynamic behavior of human brain and how it can be used to predict the arm motions.

Acknowledgements

We would like to mention the funding body, i.e. Higher Education Commission (HEC) of Pakistan who awarded the grant under NRPU project number 10702. We would also like to show gratitude to the friends who connected us with the amputees.

Author details

Usama Ali Syed*, Zareena Kausar and Neelum Yousaf Sattar
Air University, Islamabad, Pakistan

*Address all correspondence to: syed.a.usama@outlook.com

References

[1] Lobo-Prat J, Kooren PN, Stienen AH, Herder JL, Koopman BF, Veltink PH. Non-invasive control interfaces for intention detection in active movement-assistive devices. Journal of Neuroengineering and Rehabilitation. 2014;**11**(1):168

[2] Fang Y, Hettiarachchi N, Zhou D, Liu H. Multi-modal sensing techniques for interfacing hand prostheses: A review. IEEE Sensors Journal. 2015;**15**(11):6065-6076

[3] Guo W, Sheng X, Liu H, Zhu X. Mechanomyography assisted myoelectric sensing for upper-extremity prostheses: A hybrid approach. IEEE Sensors Journal. 2017;**17**(10):3100-3108

[4] Guo W, Sheng X, Liu H, Zhu X. Toward an enhanced human–machine interface for upper-limb prosthesis control with combined EMG and NIRS signals. IEEE Transactions on Human-Machine Systems. 2017;**47**(4):564-575

[5] Reaz MB, Hussain MS, Mohd-Yasin F. Techniques of EMG signal analysis: Detection, processing, classification and applications (correction). Biological Procedures Online. 2006;**8**(1):163

[6] Batula AM, Mark J, Kim YE, Ayaz H, editors. Developing an optical brain-computer interface for humanoid robot control. In: International Conference on Augmented Cognition. Springer; 2016

[7] Coyle SM, Ward TE, Markham CM. Brain–computer interface using a simplified functional near-infrared spectroscopy system. Journal of Neural Engineering. 2007;**4**(3):219

[8] Sitaram R, Zhang H, Guan C, Thulasidas M, Hoshi Y, Ishikawa A, et al. Temporal classification of multichannel near-infrared spectroscopy signals of motor imagery for developing a brain–computer interface. NeuroImage. 2007;**34**(4):1416-1427

[9] Lambert J-H. Photometria, sive de Mensura et gradibus luminis, colorum et umbrae. sumptibus viduae E. Klett; 1760

[10] Abitan H, Bohr H, Buchhave P. Correction to the Beer-Lambert-Bouguer law for optical absorption. Applied Optics. 2008;**47**(29):5354-5357

[11] Beer A. Bestimmung der absorption des rothen lichts in farbigen flussigkeiten. Annalen der Physik. 1852;**162**:78-88

[12] Lambert JH. Lamberts Photometrie: Photometria, sive De mensura et gradibus luminus, colorum et umbrae (1760). W. Engelmann; 1892

[13] Herold F, Wiegel P, Scholkmann F, Müller NG. Applications of functional near-infrared spectroscopy (fNIRS) neuroimaging in exercise–cognition science: A systematic, methodology-focused review. Journal of Clinical Medicine. 2018;**7**(12):466

[14] Aresté N, Salgueira M. World Medical Association Declaration of Helsinki: Ethical principles for medical research involving human subjects. Journal of the American Medical Association. 2013;**310**(20):2191-2194

[15] Yanagisawa H, Dan I, Tsuzuki D, Kato M, Okamoto M, Kyutoku Y, et al. Acute moderate exercise elicits increased dorsolateral prefrontal activation and improves cognitive performance with Stroop test. NeuroImage. 2010;**50**(4):1702-1710

[16] Hyodo K, Dan I, Suwabe K, Kyutoku Y, Yamada Y, Akahori M, et al. Acute moderate exercise enhances compensatory brain activation in older adults. Neurobiology of Aging. 2012;**33**(11):2621-2632

[17] Byun K, Hyodo K, Suwabe K, Ochi G, Sakairi Y, Kato M, et al. Positive

effect of acute mild exercise on executive function via arousal-related prefrontal activations: An fNIRS study. NeuroImage. 2014;**98**:336-345

[18] Dupuy O, Gauthier CJ, Fraser SA, Desjardins-Crepeau L, Desjardins M, Mekary S, et al. Higher levels of cardiovascular fitness are associated with better executive function and prefrontal oxygenation in younger and older women. Frontiers in Human Neuroscience. 2015;**9**:66

[19] Hyodo K, Dan I, Kyutoku Y, Suwabe K, Byun K, Ochi G, et al. The association between aerobic fitness and cognitive function in older men mediated by frontal lateralization. NeuroImage. 2016;**125**:291-300

[20] Albinet CT, Mandrick K, Bernard PL, Perrey S, Blain H. Improved cerebral oxygenation response and executive performance as a function of cardiorespiratory fitness in older women: A fNIRS study. Frontiers in Aging Neuroscience. 2014;**6**:272

[21] Hyodo K, Suwabe K, Soya H, Nagamatsu T. The effect of an acute bout of slow aerobic dance on mood and executive function in older adults: A pilot study. Bulletin of the Physical Fitness Research Institute. 2017;**115**:35-41

[22] Wang W, Qiu C, Ota T, Sawada M, Kishimoto N, Kishimoto T. Effects of Tai Chi exercise on attention in healthy elderly subjects as measured by near-infrared spectroscopy during the Stroop task. Journal of Nara Medical Association. 2013;**64**(5):79-86

[23] Faulkner J, Stoner L, Grigg R, Fryer S, Stone K, Lambrick D. Acute effects of exercise posture on executive function in transient ischemic attack patients. Psychophysiology. 2017;**54**(8):1239-1248

[24] Moriya M, Aoki C, Sakatani K. Effects of physical exercise on working memory and prefrontal cortex function in post-stroke patients. In: Oxygen Transport to Tissue XXXVIII. Springer; 2016. pp. 203-208

[25] Tsujii T, Komatsu K, Sakatani K. Acute effects of physical exercise on prefrontal cortex activity in older adults: A functional near-infrared spectroscopy study. In: Oxygen Transport to Tissue XXXIV. Springer; 2013. pp. 293-298

[26] Liao LD, Tsytsarev V, Delgado-Martinez I, Li ML, Erzurumlu R, Vipin A, et al. Neurovascular coupling: In vivo optical techniques for functional brain imaging. Biomedical Engineering Online. 2013;**12**(1):38

[27] Chen T, Yue GH, Tian Y, Jiang C. Baduanjin mind-body intervention improves the executive control function. Frontiers in Psychology. 2016;**7**:2015

[28] Mücke M, Andrä C, Gerber M, Pühse U, Ludyga S. Moderate-to-vigorous physical activity, executive functions and prefrontal brain oxygenation in children: A functional near-infrared spectroscopy study. Journal of Sports Sciences. 2018;**36**(6):630-636

[29] Kato K, Iwamoto K, Kawano N, Noda Y, Ozaki N, Noda A. Differential effects of physical activity and sleep duration on cognitive function in young adults. Journal of Sport and Health Science. 2018;**7**(2):227-236

[30] Sudo M, Komiyama T, Aoyagi R, Nagamatsu T, Higaki Y, Ando S. Executive function after exhaustive exercise. European Journal of Applied Physiology. 2017;**117**(10):2029-2038

[31] Matsuda K, Ikeda S, Mitsutake T, Nakahara M, Nagai Y, Ikeda T, et al. Factors influencing executive function by physical activity level among young adults: A near-infrared spectroscopy study. Journal of Physical Therapy Science. 2017;**29**(3):470-475

[32] Makizako H, Doi T, Shimada H, Park H, Uemura K, Yoshida D, et al. Relationship between going outdoors daily and activation of the prefrontal cortex during verbal fluency tasks (VFTs) among older adults: A near-infrared spectroscopy study. Archives of Gerontology and Geriatrics. 2013;**56**(1):118-123

[33] Kujach S, Byun K, Hyodo K, Suwabe K, Fukuie T, Laskowski R, et al. A transferable high-intensity intermittent exercise improves executive performance in association with dorsolateral prefrontal activation in young adults. NeuroImage. 2018;**169**:117-125

[34] Giles GE, Cantelon JA, Eddy MD, Brunyé TT, Urry HL, Mahoney CR, et al. Habitual exercise is associated with cognitive control and cognitive reappraisal success. Experimental Brain Research. 2017;**235**(12):3785-3797

[35] Yamazaki Y, Sato D, Yamashiro K, Tsubaki A, Yamaguchi Y, Takehara N, et al. Inter-individual differences in exercise-induced spatial working memory improvement: A near-infrared spectroscopy study. In: Oxygen Transport to Tissue XXXIX. Springer; 2017. pp. 81-88

[36] Lambrick D, Stoner L, Grigg R, Faulkner J. Effects of continuous and intermittent exercise on executive function in children aged 8-10 years. Psychophysiology. 2016;**53**(9):1335-1342

[37] Quaresima V, Ferrari M. Functional near-infrared spectroscopy (fNIRS) for assessing cerebral cortex function during human behavior in natural/social situations: A concise review. Organizational Research Methods. 2019;**22**(1):46-68

[38] Perrey S. Non-invasive NIR spectroscopy of human brain function during exercise. Methods. 2008;**45**(4):289-299

[39] Pinti P, Aichelburg C, Gilbert S, Hamilton A, Hirsch J, Burgess P, et al. A review on the use of wearable functional near-infrared spectroscopy in naturalistic environments. Japanese Psychological Research. 2018;**60**(4):347-373

[40] Holtzer R, Mahoney JR, Izzetoglu M, Wang C, England S, Verghese J. Online fronto-cortical control of simple and attention-demanding locomotion in humans. NeuroImage. 2015;**112**:152-159

[41] Holtzer R, Verghese J, Allali G, Izzetoglu M, Wang C, Mahoney JR. Neurological gait abnormalities moderate the functional brain signature of the posture first hypothesis. Brain Topography. 2016;**29**(2):334-343

[42] Cui X, Bray S, Reiss AL. Speeded near infrared spectroscopy (NIRS) response detection. PLoS One. 2010;**5**(11):e15474

[43] Strangman G, Boas DA, Sutton JP. Non-invasive neuroimaging using near-infrared light. Biological Psychiatry. 2002;**52**(7):679-693

[44] Strangman G, Franceschini MA, Boas DA. Factors affecting the accuracy of near-infrared spectroscopy concentration calculations for focal changes in oxygenation parameters. NeuroImage. 2003;**18**(4):865-879

[45] Scholkmann F, Spichtig S, Muehlemann T, Wolf M. How to detect and reduce movement artifacts in near-infrared imaging using moving standard deviation and spline interpolation. Physiological Measurement. 2010;**31**(5):649

[46] Scholkmann F, Wolf M. Measuring brain activity using functional near infrared spectroscopy: A short review. Spectroscopy Europe. 2012;**24**(4):6

[47] Ando S, Yamada Y, Kokubu M. Reaction time to peripheral visual

stimuli during exercise under hypoxia. Journal of Applied Physiology. 2010;**108**(5):1210-1216

[48] Villringer A, Chance B. Non-invasive optical spectroscopy and imaging of human brain function. Trends in Neurosciences. 1997;**20**(10):435-442

[49] Issard C, Gervain J. Variability of the hemodynamic response in infants: Influence of experimental design and stimulus complexity. Developmental Cognitive Neuroscience. 2018;**33**:182-193

[50] Demandt E, Mehring C, Vogt K, Schulze-Bonhage A, Aertsen A, Ball T. Reaching movement onset-and end-related characteristics of EEG spectral power modulations. Frontiers in Neuroscience. 2012;**6**:65

[51] Herold F, Wiegel P, Scholkmann F, Thiers A, Hamacher D, Schega L. Functional near-infrared spectroscopy in movement science: A systematic review on cortical activity in postural and walking tasks. Neurophotonics. 2017;**4**(4):041403

Chapter 5

Flicker-Noise Spectroscopy Method in the Problem of Diagnosing the State of the Cardiovascular System

Abdullayev Namiq Tahir and Ahmadova Khadija Ramiz

Abstract

In the field of research of the cardiovascular system, mainly analysis methods that are strictly mathematically applicable to stationary signals are distinguished; however, nonstationary signals prevail in medical practice, the statistical properties of which vary with time. Often they consist of short-term high-frequency components, followed by long-term low-frequency components. Given this nature of bioelectric potentials, and in particular electrocardiographic signals, the most suitable for their analysis may be the nonlinear dynamics method with the calculation of quantitative characteristics of chaos. This possibility is presented by the flicker-noise spectroscopy method, which takes into account the intermittency effect in a complex dynamic system when sections of chaotic bursts and jumps alternate with relatively long sections of a laminar nature. The analysis of signals of such a dynamic nature is usually based on the use of flicker-noise spectroscopy.

Keywords: flicker-noise spectroscopy, electrocardiographic signals, analysis, intermittency, diagnostics

1. Introduction

The flicker-noise spectroscopy method is proposed as a general phenomenological (non-model) approach to the analysis of chaotic signals of different nature. The essence of flicker-noise spectroscopy is to give informational significance to the correlation relationships that are realized in sequences of signal irregularities—bursts, jumps, and kinks of derivatives of various orders—as carriers of information about changes occurring at each spatiotemporal level of the hierarchical organization of the dynamic system under study. The autocorrelation function $\psi(\tau)$ is used as a basic image for extracting information from complex signals in the flicker-noise spectroscopy method [1, 2].

To classify information, this function is not analyzed but some of its transformations ("projections"), such as power spectrum $S(f)$, where f is the signal frequency, and the difference moment ("transition structure function") $\Phi^{(2)}(\tau)$ of the second order. The information extracted from the analysis of dependencies $S(f)$ and $\Phi^{(2)}(\tau)$, built on the basis of time series $V(t)$, has the meaning of correlation times or parameters, characterizing the loss of correlation relationships ("memory") for the irregularities under consideration such as bursts and jumps.

Moreover, only irregularities of the type of jumps of dynamic variable $V(t)$ contribute to the formation of dependence $\Phi^{(2)}(\tau)$, and jumps and bursts (outbursts) of chaotic series $V(t)$ contribute to the formation of $S(f)$.

The solution to the problem of predicting the evolution of a complex system and, above all, the search for precursors (precursors) of catastrophic changes in it is associated with the most dramatic changes in dependencies $S(f)$ and $\Phi^{(2)}(\tau)$ ($p = 2, 3, \ldots$) calculated on the basis of high-frequency and low-frequency components $V(t)$.

2. Splitting an electrocardiographic signal into low-frequency and high-frequency components

The behavior of the electrocardiographic signal, reflecting the functional state of the cardiovascular system, is quite complicated and has the character of randomness.

The most general form of evolution in dynamic variable $V(t_i)$ for the ith space–time level of the electrocardiographic signal is presented in the form of intermittency, when not all intervals on the time axis are informationally equivalent. Such dynamics of the electrocardiogram (ECG) is characterized (**Figure 1**) by relatively weak changes in the variable over relatively long time intervals—"laminar phases" with characteristic durations of T_i and sudden interruptions of such evolution by abrupt changes in the value of the dynamic variable in the short intervals of duration τ_i ($\tau_i < T_i$).

Each such abrupt change in the values of a dynamic variable then ends up with values in the subsequent "laminar" section. The magnitude and duration of such jumps, surges, and "laminar" sections are specific for each of the cardiovascular systems, causing a certain contribution to the corresponding power spectrum.

In this case, the studied signal $V(t)$ is conveniently represented as the sum of the two terms: the singular term $V_S(t)$, which is formed only by bursts of the dynamic variable, and the regular term $V_R(t) = V(t) - V_S(t)$, which is formed after subtracting bursts from the presented signal and determined by the jumps of the dynamic variable and "laminar phases."

The analysis of the electrocardiogram shows that it corresponds to the described dynamics, when bursts in the form of QRS complexes alternate with rather small jumps in the form of P and T teeth and extended phases in the form of an isoline.

The information contained in $S(f)$ and $\Phi^{(2)}(\tau)$ is different, so in order to determine the adequate parameters of the structure under study, it is necessary to analyze the dependencies $\log S(f) = F(\log f)$ and $\log \Phi^{(2)}(\tau) = F(\log \tau)$.

Let $V(t)$ denotes the dynamic variable, characterizing the ECG signal. We apply the proposed method of splitting the dynamic signal into low-frequency $V_R(t)$ and

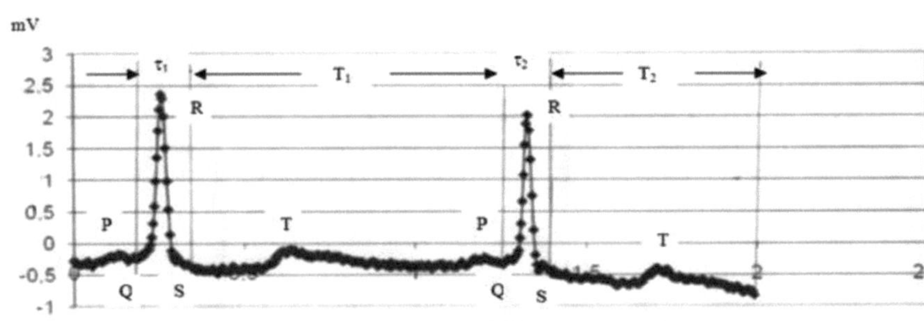

Figure 1.
The dynamics of the electrocardiogram.

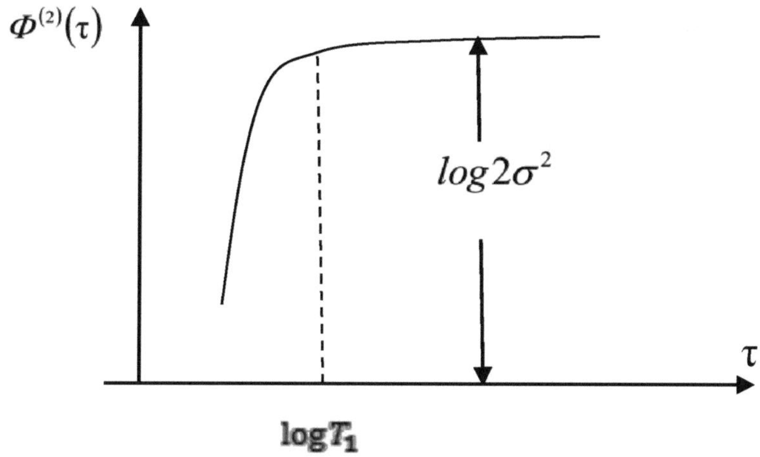

Figure 2.
Typical curve for function $\Phi^{(2)}(\tau)$, characterizing a chaotic signal $V(t)$ without a resonant component.

high-frequency $V_S(t)$ components. This method is built by analogy (**Figure 2**) with the solution of the diffusion equation and is based on the following "relaxation" procedure:

1. Set the value $V_1, \ldots, V_N$ of signal V with a step of discreteness Δt.

2. Calculate $\langle V \rangle = \frac{1}{N}\sum_{k=1}^{n} V(k)$ and put $V_{(R)} := V_{(k)} - \langle V \rangle, k = 1, \ldots, N$.

3. We calculate

$$\psi(m_\tau) = \frac{1}{N - m_\tau} \sum_{k=1}^{N-m_\tau} V_{(k)} V_{(k+m_\tau)}, \mathrm{m}_\tau = [\tau/\Delta \mathrm{t}] \tag{1}$$

where $\Phi^{(2)}(\tau) = 2[\psi(0) - \psi(\tau)], \sigma^2 = \psi(0),\ \tau = \mathrm{m}_\tau \cdot \Delta \mathrm{t}$

$$\mathrm{m}_\tau = 0, 1, \ldots, \mathrm{M} - 1, \mathrm{M} \in \mathrm{N} \tag{2}$$

4. We plot $\Phi^{(2)}(\tau)$ in bilogarithmic coordinates.

   The asymptotic representation for $\Phi^{(2)}(\tau)$ is

$$\Phi^{(2)}(\tau) = \begin{cases} \tau^{2\mathrm{H}_1}, & if\, \tau << \mathrm{T}_1 \\ 2\sigma^2, & if\, \tau >> \mathrm{T}_1. \end{cases} \tag{3}$$

5. We take for T_1 the value τ, at which $\log \Phi^{(2)}(\tau)$ begins to stabilize to a constant equal to $\log (2\sigma^2)$.

6. Choose a sequence of small $\{\tau_k\}$ ($\mathrm{k} = 1, \ldots, \mathrm{k}_0$ $\mathrm{k}_0 \approx 20$), $\tau_k << \mathrm{T}_1$, and construct a regression $\mathrm{y} = \mathrm{ax} + \mathrm{b}$ ($\mathrm{b} = 0$); $\mathrm{y} = \ln \Phi^{(2)}(\tau), \mathrm{x} = ln\, \tau, \mathrm{a} = 2\mathrm{H}_1$.

According to the least squares method (LSM) estimate $\hat{a}$, we calculate the estimate $\mathrm{H}_1 = \hat{a}/2$.

7. We calculate

$$D = \frac{\sigma^2}{\Gamma^2(1 + H_1^*) \cdot T_1^*} \tag{4}$$

To calculate $\Gamma(x)$ for $x = 1 + H_1$, put $n = 10^3$and represent $\Gamma(x)$ in the form

$$\Gamma(x) = \frac{\Gamma(x+1)}{x} = \frac{\Gamma(x+2)}{x(x+1)} = \dots = \frac{\Gamma(x+n)}{x(x+1)\cdot(x+nt)}. \tag{5}$$

The value $\Gamma(z)$ (we have $z = x + n$) is calculated by the formula

$$\Gamma(z) = exp\left\{\left(z - \frac{1}{2}\right) \ln z - z + \frac{1}{2}\, ln\, 2\pi\right\} \tag{6}$$

with an error of order $z^{-1} \approx 10^{-3}\ n \approx 10^3\ z = x + n$.

8. Denote by Δt and $\Delta\tau$ the steps of discreteness in t and τ, and

$$\omega = D \cdot \Delta\tau/(\Delta t)^2 \tag{7}$$

choose $\Delta\tau$ so that $\omega < 1/2$.

9. Put $M := N - 1$, and construct an iterative procedure according to $j = 0, 1, \dots,$, according to which the value V_k^{j+1} at the jth step is calculated through the value V_k^j according to the formula

$$V_k^{j+1} = \omega V_{k+1}^j + \omega V_{k\text{-}1}^j + (1 - 2\omega)\, V_k^j \tag{8}$$

at $j = 0$ we set $V_k^j = V_{(k)}$; at $k = 1$ and $k = M$, the values of $V_k^{j+1}$are calculated by the formulas

$$V_1^{j+1} = (1 - 2\omega)\, V_1^j + 2\omega V_2^j, \quad V_M^{j+1} = (1 - 2\omega)\, V_M^j + 2\omega V_{M-1}^j. \tag{9}$$

The procedure stops at step $j = j_0$, in which.

$$\left|V_k^{j_0+1} - V_k^{j_0}\right| < \varepsilon, \text{ for } V_k = 1, \dots, M, k = 1, 2, \dots, N,$$

where ε is the given number (e.g., $\varepsilon = 10^{-m+1}$, where $10^{-m}$is the error in setting the initial values V_k).

10. The values $V_k^{j_0}$ determine the low-frequency component $V_R(t)$. Then $V(t) - V_R(t) = V_S(t)$ is the high-frequency component of the signal $V(t)$.

The described signal smoothing procedure is focused on minimizing the "high-frequency" information in the "low-frequency" part $V_R(t)$ of the signal and vice versa, minimizing the "low-frequency" information in the "high-frequency" part $V_S(t)$ of the signal. This conclusion follows from the diffusion nature of the partial differential equation used

$$\frac{\partial V}{\partial \tau} = \frac{\partial^2 V}{\partial t^2}, \tag{10}$$

represented as a difference equation

$$\frac{V_k^{j+1} - V_k^j}{\Delta\tau} = \frac{V_{k+1}^j + V_{k-1}^j - 2V_k^j}{(\Delta t)^2}, \tag{11}$$

corresponding to the simplest difference scheme for numerically solving Eq. (10). From (11) we obtain

$$V_k^{j+1} = V_k^j + \frac{\Delta\tau}{(\Delta t)^2}\left(V_{k+1}^j + V_{k-1}^j - 2V_k^j\right).$$

In notation $\omega = \Delta\tau/(\Delta t)^2$, the last equation is written in the form (8). From the theory of stability of difference schemes, it is known that this difference scheme will be absolutely stable at $\omega < 1/2$.

Such a relaxation procedure realizes the maximum rate of entropy generation and uses the relationship of entropy and Fisher information, which is a quantitative measure of the heterogeneity of the distribution density of the analyzed data array.

3. Parameterization of the singular component of the ECG signal

The procedure for parameterizing the singular part of the signal consists of the following sequence of steps [3]:

1. Let V(t) be represented as a sum

$$V(t) = V_R(t) + V_S(t).$$

2. Let $t_k = k\Delta t (k = 1, \dots, N), t_0 = 0, t_N = T$ points of task $V(t)$ by $[0, T]$ with a certain step of discreteness $\Delta t; N = [T/\Delta t]$.

   We calculate the average value:

$$\langle V(t)\rangle = \frac{1}{N}\sum_{k=1}^{N} V(t_k) \tag{12}$$

   In what follows, we will assume that $\langle V(t)\rangle = 0$, i.e., signal $V(t)$, is stationary.

3. For stationary signal $V(t)$, the power spectrum $S(f)$ (Fourier transform of the autocorrelation function $\psi(\tau)$) coincides with $S_c(f)$ (cosine Fourier transform of $\psi(\tau)$).

   We set M from condition $\frac{4}{3} \le M \le N$ (in practice, take M close to N). We assume that M is an even number. For a time delay of $m_\tau = 0, 1, \dots, M-1$, we calculate the autocorrelator:

$$\psi(m_\tau) = \frac{1}{N - m_\tau}\sum_{k=1}^{N-m_\tau} V(k)V(k + m_\tau) \tag{13}$$

4. Let $f = \frac{q/M}{\Delta t}$.

   We calculate the power spectrum $S(f) = S_c(f)$

$$S_c(f) = \frac{1}{\Delta t} S_c(q)$$

$$S_c(q) = \psi(0) + \psi\left(\frac{M}{2}\right)(-1)^q + 2\sum_{m=1}^{\frac{M}{2}-1} \psi(m)\cos\left(\frac{2\pi q m}{M}\right), \tag{14}$$

$$(q = 0, 1, \dots, M-1)$$

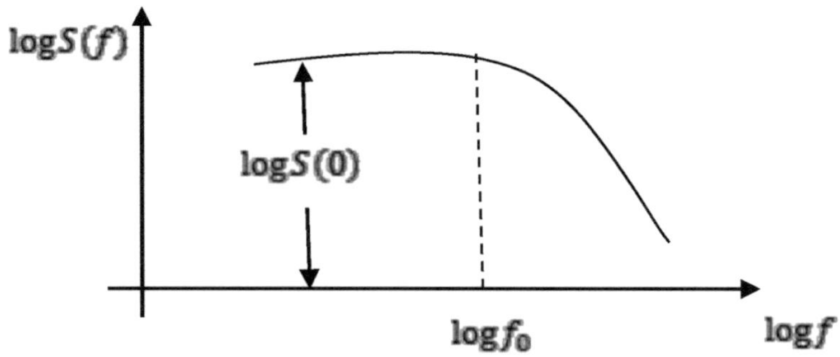

Figure 3.
Typical curve for function $S(f)$, characterizing a chaotic signal $V(t)$ without a resonant component.

5. We will construct the image $S(f)$ (or $|S(f)|$, if in some frequencies $S(f) < 0$) in a bilogarithmic scale (**Figure 3**).

   From **Figure 3** we find the frequency $f = f_0$, starting from which $S(f)$ ceases to stabilize around a certain constant $S(0)$.

6. Let $\left[f^*, \overline{f}^*\right]$ be the frequency interval in the region of the graph $S(f)$ (or $|S(f)|$), preceding the first strong peak of the power spectrum $S(f)$, corresponding to "irregularity-burst." We assume that $S(f)$ increases at $f \in \left[f^*, \overline{f}^*\right]$ and $S_s^*(0)$—a certain number from interval $\left[S(f^*), S\left(\overline{f}^*\right)\right]$.

7. We calculate the autocorrelator $\psi_{S,R}(\tau)$ according to the formula.

$$\psi_{S,R}(\tau) = \frac{1}{N - m_\tau} \sum_{k=1}^{N-m_\tau} [V_S(k)V_S(k+m_\tau) + V_R(k)V_S(k+m_\tau) + V_S(k)V_R(k+m_\tau)],$$
$$(m_\tau = 0, 1, \dots, M-1) \tag{15}$$

8. We calculate the singular component $S_S(f)$ of spectrum $S(f)$ by the formula

$$S_S(f) = \frac{1}{\Delta t} S_S(q)$$
$$S_S(q) = \psi_{S,R}(0) + \psi_{S,R}\left(\frac{M}{2}\right)(-1)^q + 2 \sum_{m=1}^{\frac{M}{2}-1} \psi_{S,R}(m) \cos\left(\frac{2\pi q m}{M}\right) \tag{16}$$
$$(q = 0, 1, \dots, M-1)$$

9. For parameterization $S_S(f)$, we approximate this function by an interpolation expression:

$$\hat{S}_S(f) \approx \frac{S_S(0)}{1 + (2\pi f T_0)^{n_0}} \tag{17}$$

   Parameter T_0 by formula (17) will be determined by **Algorithm 1**, assuming that the "experimental" spectrum $S_S(f)$ is calculated by formula (16).

Algorithm 1.

9.1. Using the spectrum graph (**Figure 3**), we introduce the constants $f_0^*, \underline{f}^*, \overline{f}^*, S_S^*(0)$, as well as the threshold value $RSS^* = 10^{10}$.
9.2. We set $S_S(0) = S_S^*(0)$ and evaluate the parameters T_0, n_0.
Build a regression

$$y = ax + b,$$

where

$$y = \ln\left|\frac{S_s(0)}{S_s(f)} - 1\right|, x = \ln 2\pi f, a = n_0, b = n_0 \ln T_0,$$

and estimate the coefficients a and b using the least squares method (least squares) for sample $\{y_m, x_m\}$ with y_m and x_m, corresponding to frequencies $f_m = \frac{m}{M \cdot \Delta t}$ $(m = 0, 1, \dots, M-1)$.
We calculate the residual sum of squares

$$RSS^{(1)} = \sum_{m=0}^{M-1}\left[y_m - \left(\hat{a}x_m + \hat{b}\right)\right]^2,$$

where $\hat{a}$ and $\hat{b}$ LSM are the estimations of parameters a and b.
If $RSS^{(1)} < RSS^*$, then $RSS^* := RSS^{(1)}$, $\hat{n}_0 = n_0^*$, $T_0^* = \hat{T}_0$, where $\hat{n}_0 = \hat{a}$, $\hat{T}_0 = exp\left\{\hat{b}/\hat{a}\right\}$.
9.3. We set $n_0 = n_0^*$, $S_S(0) = S_S^*(0)$and evaluate T_0.
Build a regression

$$y = ax + b(b = 0),$$

where

$$y = \left|\frac{S_s(0)}{S_s(f)} - 1\right|^{1/n_0}, x = 2\pi f, a = T_0.$$

We calculate $RSS^{(2)} = \sum_{m=0}^{M-1}\left[y_m - \hat{a}x_m\right]^2$.
If $RSS^{(2)} < RSS^*$, then $RSS^* := RSS^{(2)}$ and $T_0^* = \hat{T}_0$, where $\hat{T}_0 = \hat{a}$.
9.4. We set $T_0 = T_0^*$, $n_0 = n_0^*$ and evaluate $S_S(0)$.
Build a regression

$$y = ax + b(b = 0),$$

where

$$y = S_s(f), x = \frac{1}{1 + (2\pi f\, T_0)\, n_0}, \quad a = S_S(0)$$

We calculate $RSS^{(3)} = \sum_{m=0}^{M-1}\left[y_m - \hat{a}x_m\right]^2$.
If $RSS^{(3)} < RSS^*$, then $RSS^* := RSS^{(3)}$, $S_S(0) = \hat{S}_S(0)$, where $\hat{S}_S(0) = \hat{a}$.
9.5. We set $S_S(0) = S_S^*(0)$, $T_0 = T_0^*$ and evaluate n_0.

Build a regression

$$y = ax + b(b = 0),$$

where

$$y = ln\left|\frac{S_s(0)}{S_s(f)} - 1\right|, x = ln\,(2\pi f T_0), a = n_0.$$

We calculate $RSS^{(4)} = \sum_{m=0}^{M-1} \left[y_m - \hat{a}x_m\right]^2$.

If $RSS^{(4)} < RSS^*$, then $n_0^* = \hat{n}_0$, where $\hat{n}_0 = \hat{a}$.

As a result of **Algorithm 1**, we obtain the three parameters $S_S(0) = S_S^*(0)$, $n_0 = n_0^*$, $T_0 = T_0^*$, characterizing the interpolation expression (17) for the singular component of the spectrum $S_S(f)$.

4. Informative diagnostic parameters of the singular component of the ECG signal

During a computational experiment, electrocardiographic signals with a normal state of the cardiovascular system and pathological signals ("tachycardia," "arrhythmia," and "atrial fibrillation") were analyzed. We used data from the public site www.PhysioNet.org for the II standard lead. The ECG removal parameters (type of lead, sampling frequency, time, number of samples, and signal amplitude) are included in the sample. The sampling rate for various samples varies from 125 to 1000 Hz. The values of the presented samples, taking into account the sign discharge, correspond to the use of a 12-bit ADC.

In **Figures 4–6**, the graphs of the spectral power of the ECG signal for the norm, the singular component of this signal, and the estimation of the singular component of this signal are presented.

In **Figures 7–9**, as an example, similar relationships for an ECG signal with a range of "atrial arrhythmia" are presented.

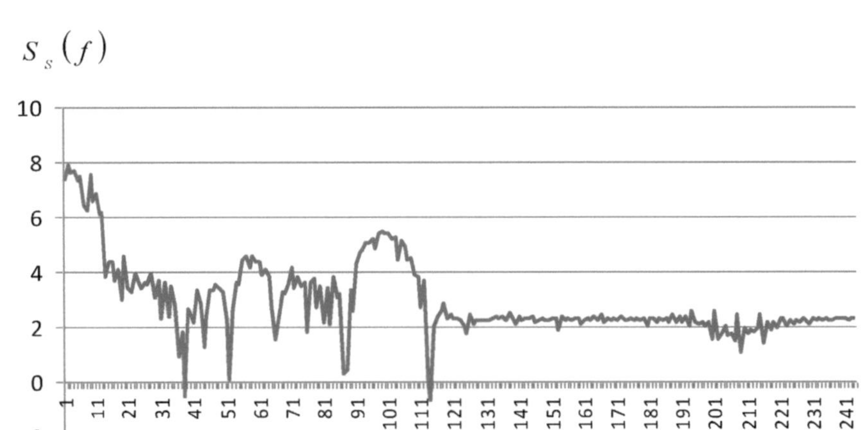

Figure 4.
Graphs of the spectral power of the ECG signal for the norm.

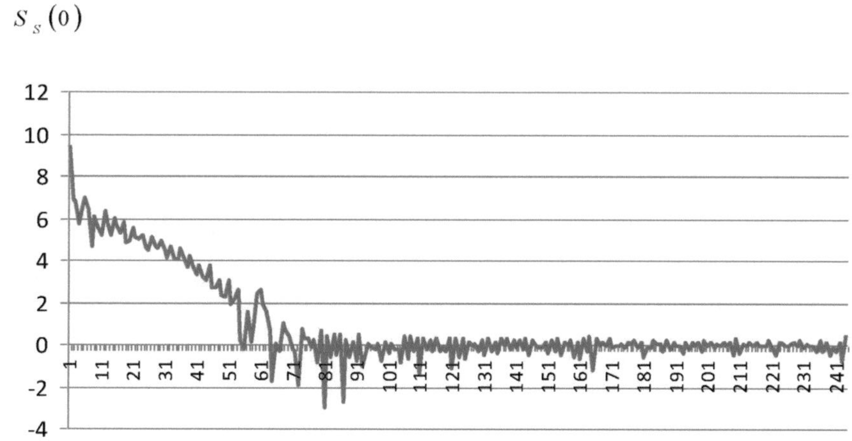

Figure 5.
Graphs of the singular component of this signal.

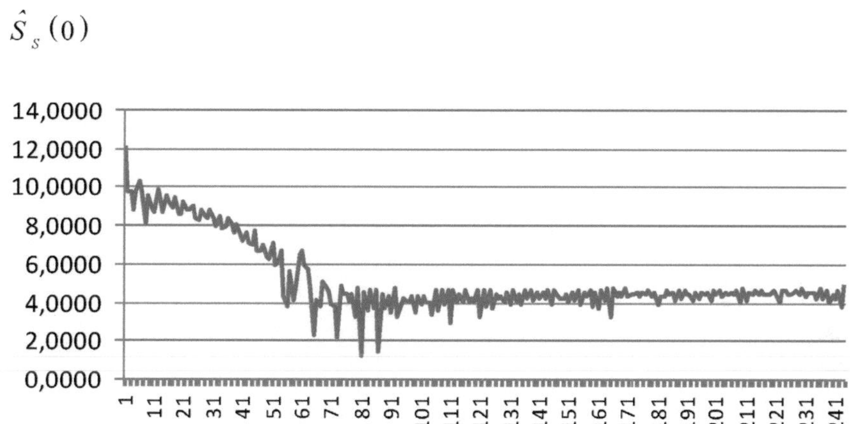

Figure 6.
Graphs of the estimation of the singular component of this signal.

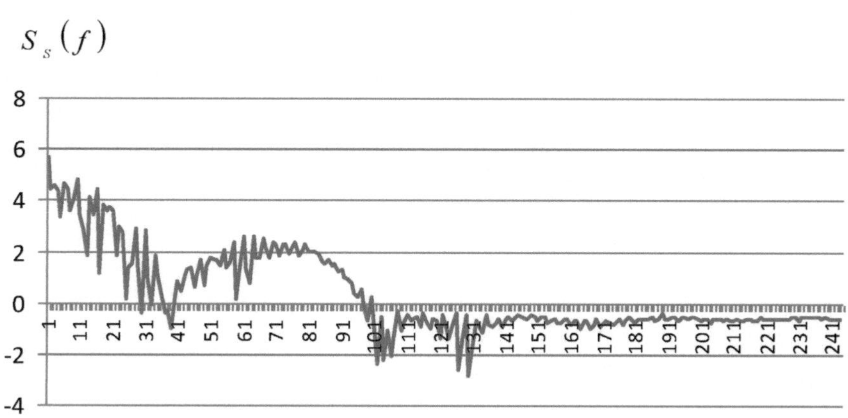

Figure 7.
Graphs of the spectral power of the ECG signal for the "atrial arrhythmia."

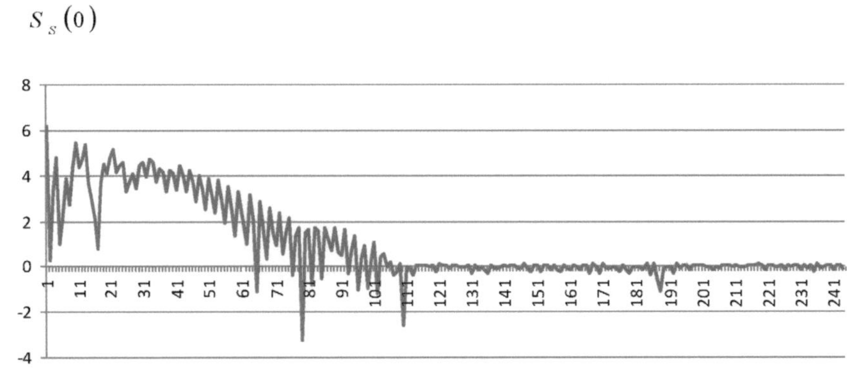

Figure 8.
Graphs of the singular component of the "atrial arrhythmia."

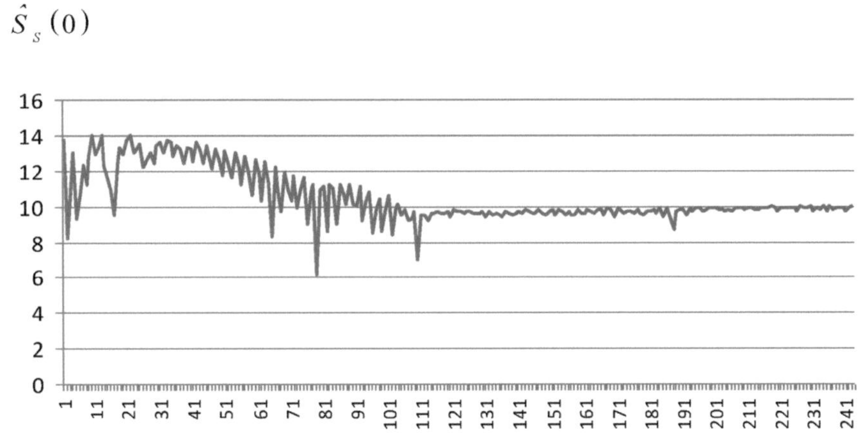

Figure 9.
Graphs of the estimation of the singular component of the "atrial arrhythmia."

For all the considered states of the cardiovascular system, the same dependencies were obtained, and based on the obtained dependencies, informative parameters of the singular component of the ECG signals were calculated (**Table 1**).

The high specificity of $S(f)$ patterns obtained in the study of the cardiovascular system in the norm with the indicated pathologies can be used to diagnose diseases. Dependence $S(f)$ built on the basis of different ECGs and the corresponding informative parameters obtained by them differ from each other, which gives

ECG signal	n_0	T_0	$S_s(0)$
Norm	0.3414	0.0042	437.8090
Atrial fibrillation	0.3836	0.0036	334.3640
Ventricular tachycardia	0.4123	0.0032	197.3580
Atrial arrhythmia	0.4013	0.0059	43.7105

Table 1.
Informative parameters of the singular component of ECG signals.

reason to consider these dependencies as patterns characterizing the condition of the patient under study. The obtained informative parameters can be considered as distinguishing features for the differential diagnosis of cardiovascular diseases (e.g., using artificial neural networks).

This approach shows the possibility of flicker-noise spectroscopy as a method that allows you to establish significant differences in the original, visually not very different, ECG signals.

5. Parameterization of the regular part of the ECG signal and determination of informative diagnostic parameters

The determination of the parameters of a chaotic signal given on a limited interval T is set on the basis of the flicker-noise spectroscopy method, taking into account the contributions of the "resonant components" to the autocorrelation function [4].

$$\Psi(\tau) = \langle V(t), V(t+\tau) \rangle, \tag{18}$$

and, therefore, to cosine conversion

$$S_c(f) = \int_{-T/2}^{T/2} \Psi(\tau) \cos(2\pi f \tau) d\tau \tag{19}$$

and second-order difference moment

$$\Phi^{(2)}(\tau) = \left\langle |V(t) - V(t+\tau|^2 \right\rangle. \tag{20}$$

Here $V(t)$ is a stationary signal ($\langle V(t) \rangle = 0$), and $\langle \cdot \rangle$ is a symbol of the average value.

The developed method of signal parametrization is based on the fact that the introduced "irregularities-bursts" and "irregularities-jumps" contribute to various spectral regions of dependence $S(f)$.

In fact, the first step in the parameterization of irregularities was to isolate the "burst" (singular), most "high-frequency" (the so-called "flicker-noise tail") component of the signal irregularities in the spectral dependence $S(f)$.

Based on the remaining (after subtracting the "burst" contribution) spectral dependence, we can now determine the structure function $\Phi^{(2)}(\tau)$, which contains the contributions from the "jump" and "resonance" components that slowly change against its background. The next steps are to parameterize the "higher frequency" (of those remaining) "hopping" (regular) component using the least squares method.

It must be borne in mind that when solving the signal parametrization problem under consideration, problems arise due to the limited averaging interval T. For this reason, in particular, it is the "experimental" dependence $V(t)$ constructed on the basis of observed signal $S(f)$ that may turn out to be negative in some frequency intervals. Therefore along with four in such cases, $S(f)$ is introduced into consideration.

The procedure for parameterizing the regular part of the signal is presented below in the form of the following sequence of operations:

1. From the extreme spectrum $S(f)$, we subtract the singular component $S_s(f)$ calculated by the interpolation formula (we denote the result by $S_{rR}(f)$)

$$S_{rR}(f) = S(f) - S_s(f) \tag{21}$$

The resulting difference characterizes the contribution of the "resonant" components $S_r(f)$ and the "irregularities-jumps" $S_R(f)$ to the general dependence $S(f)$. If it turns out that $S_{rR}(f) < 0$ in some frequency intervals, we assume $S_{rR}(f) := |S_{rR}(f)|$.

2. Take the inverse cosine Fourier transform of $S_{rR}(f)$

$$\psi_{rR}(\tau) = 2\int_0^{f_{max}} S(f)\cos(2\pi f\tau)df, (\tau \le \tau^* = T/4) \tag{22}$$

$$f_{max} = \frac{1}{4\Delta t}, \tau = k\cdot\Delta\tau(k = 1, \ldots, k_0), \Delta\tau = \frac{T/4}{k_0}, k_0 = 500.$$

Put $a = 0, b = f_{max}, h = f_{max}/n, n = 100$, $S_{rR}(f)\cdot\cos(2\pi f\tau) = g(f, \tau)$ and apply the trapezoid formula:

$$\int_a^b g(f,\tau)df = h\left(\frac{g(a,\tau)}{2} + g(a+h,\tau) + g(a+2h,\tau) + \ldots + g(b-h,\tau) + \frac{g(b,\tau)}{2}\right)$$

3. We calculate

$$\Phi_{rR}^{(2)}(\tau) = 2[\psi_{rR}(0) - \psi_{rR}(\tau)], \tau = k\cdot\Delta\tau(k = 1, \ldots, k_0)$$

4. Put $\tilde{\Phi}_r^{(2)}(\tau) = \tilde{\Phi}_{rR}^{(2)}(\tau)$.
5. We denote

$$\tilde{\Phi}^{(2)}(\tau) = \Phi_r^{(2)}(\tau) + \Phi_R^{(2)}(\tau). \tag{23}$$

where $\Phi_R^{(2)}(\tau)$ is given by the interpolation formula:

$$\Phi_R^{(2)}(\tau) = \begin{cases} 2\sigma_1^2\cdot\dfrac{1}{\Gamma^2(H_1+1)}\left(\dfrac{\tau}{T_1}\right)^{2H_1}, \tau << T_1, \\ 2\sigma_1^2\left[1 - \Gamma^{-1}(H_1)\left(\frac{\tau}{T_1}\right)^{H_1-1} exp\left(-\frac{\tau}{T_1}\right)\right]^2 \end{cases} \tag{24}$$

6. Compare the experimental structural function $\Phi^{(2)}(\tau)$, determined by the formula

$$\Phi^{(2)}(\tau) = 2[\psi(0) - \psi(\tau)], \tag{25}$$

where

$$\psi(m_\tau) = \frac{1}{N - m_\tau}\sum_{k=1}^{N-m_\tau} V_{(k)}V_{(k+m_\tau)} \qquad m_\tau = [\tau/\Delta t] \tag{26}$$

with function $\Phi^{(2)}(\tau)$ determined by formula (20) using the least squares method.

- We set $RSS^* = 10^{10}$, $T_1 = T_1^*$
- A preliminary estimate T_1^* of parameter T_1 can be obtained using the asymptotic representation of structure function $\Phi^{(2)}(\tau)$ (**Figure 10**).

The value $\Phi^{(2)}(\tau)$ is taken as T_1^* for small delays, at which $\Phi^{(2)}(\tau) \approx 2\sigma^2$ takes the maximum value $\Phi^{(2)}(\tau) \approx 2\sigma^2$.
We estimate parameters σ_1, H_1 at $\tau < < T_1$.
Build a regression

$$y = ax + b,$$

where

$$y = \ln\left\{\Phi^{(2)}(\tau) - \Phi_r^{(2)}\right\}, x = \ln\left\{\frac{\tau}{\tau_1}\right\}, a = 2H_1, b = 2\ln\frac{\sigma_1}{\Gamma^2(H_1+1)}.$$

LSM-estimates $\hat{a}$ and $\hat{b}$ are obtained on the basis of sequence $\{\tau_k\}$, $(k = 1, \dots, k_1)$ close to $\tau = 0$, using representation (21) for $\hat{\Phi}^{(2)}(\tau)$.
We calculate

$$\mathrm{RSS}^{(1)} = \sum_{k=1}^{k_1} \left[\mathrm{y}_k - (\hat{\mathrm{a}}\mathrm{x}_k + \mathrm{b})\right]^2,$$

- where y_k and x_k correspond to delays τ_k.
- If $RSS^{(1)} \geq RSS^*$, then go to Section 6.5.
- Otherwise, set $RSS^* := RSS^{(1)}$, $\sigma_1^* = \hat{\sigma}_1$, and $\mathrm{H}_1^* = \hat{H}_1$, where $\hat{\mathrm{H}}_1 = \frac{\hat{a}}{2}$ and $\hat{\sigma}_1 = \Gamma^2(\hat{H}_1 + 1)\exp\left\{\hat{b}/2\right\}$.

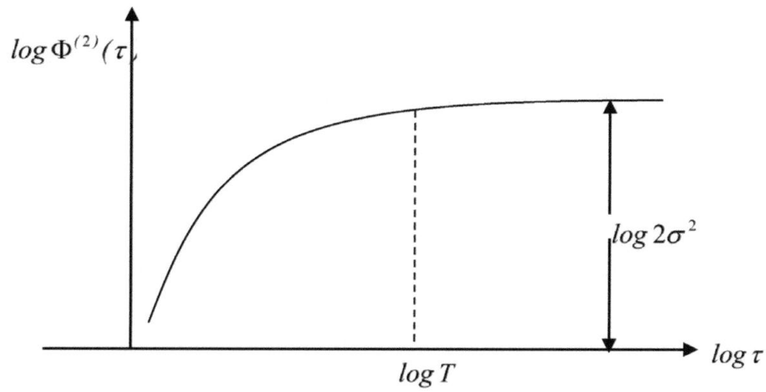

Figure 10.
Graph of function $\Phi^{(2)}(\tau)$ in bilogarithmic coordinates.

- Given $\sigma_1 = \sigma_1^*$, we estimate H_1, T_1 at $\tau << T_1$
- Build a regression

$$y = ax + b(b \neq 0),$$

- where $a = 2H_1, b = -\ln\Gamma^2(H_1+1) - 2H_1 \ln T_1, y = \ln\left\{\frac{\Phi^{(2)}(\tau) - \Phi_r^{(2)}}{2\sigma_1^2}\right\}, x = \ln\tau.$
- LSM grades $\hat{a}$ and $\hat{b}$ are obtained by sequence $\{\tau_k\}, (k = 1, \dots, k_1)$.
- We calculate

$$RSS^{(2)} = \sum_{k=1}^{k_1}\left[y_k - \left(\hat{a}x_k + \hat{b}\right)\right].$$

- If $RSS^{(2)} \geq RSS^*$, then go to Section 6.5.
- Otherwise, set $H_1^* = \hat{H}_1, T_1^* = \hat{T}_1$, where $\hat{H}_1 = \frac{\hat{a}}{2}, \hat{T}_1 = \{\Gamma^2(H_1+1)\}^{-\frac{1}{2H_1}} \exp\left\{-\frac{b}{2H_1}\right\}.$
- Given $\sigma_1 = \sigma_1^*, H_1 = H_1^*$, we estimate T_1 at $\tau << T_1$.
- Build a regression

$$y = ax + b(b = 0),$$

where

$$y = \ln\left\{\frac{\Phi^{(2)}(\tau) - \Phi_r^{(2)}(\tau)}{2\sigma_1^2/\Gamma^2(H_1+1)}\right\}, x = \tau, a = \frac{1}{T_1}.$$

- In LSM, a score of $\hat{a}$ will be obtained by sequence $\{\tau_k\}$, $(k = 1, \dots, k_1,\ k_1 << k_0)$.
- We calculate $T_1 = 1/\hat{a}$
- We calculate $RSS^{(3)} = \sum_{k=1}^{k_1}\left[y_k - \hat{a}x_k\right]^2$.
- If $RSS^{(3)} \geq RSS^*$, then go to Section 6.5.
- Otherwise, we set $RSS^* = RSS^{(3)}, T_1^* = \hat{T}_1$.
- Given $H_1 = H_1^*, T_1 = T_1^*$, we estimate σ_1 at $\tau >> T_1$.
- Build a regression

$$y = ax + b(b = 0),$$

- where $y = \Phi^{(2)}(\tau) - \Phi_r^{(2)}$, $x = \left[1 - \Gamma^{-1}(H_1)\left(\frac{\tau}{T_1}\right)^{H_1-1} \exp\left\{-\frac{\tau}{T_1}\right\}\right]^2$, $a = 2\sigma_1$.
- We calculate the least squares method (LSM) estimation by sequence $\{\tau_k\}$, $\tau_k = T - k\ \ (k = 1, \ldots, k_1)$.
- We calculate $\hat{\sigma}_1 = \sqrt{\hat{a}/2}$.
- We calculate $RSS^{(4)} = \sum_{k=1}^{k_1} (\mathrm{y}_k - \hat{\mathrm{a}}\mathrm{x}_k)^2$.
- If $RSS^{(4)} > > RSS^*$, then go to Section 6.5.
- Otherwise, we set $RSS^* = RSS^{(4)}$, $\sigma_1^* = \hat{\sigma}_1$.
- 6.5. Suppose RSS^*, σ_1^*, H_1^*, T_1^*.
- As a result of the proposed algorithm, we obtain the three parameters $\sigma_1 = \sigma_1^*$, $H_1 = H_1^*$, and $T_1 = T_1^*$, characterizing the interpolation expression (21) for $\Phi_R^{(2)}(\tau)$.

6. Informative diagnostic parameters of the regular component of the ECG signal

Using the above algorithm, we obtained the graphs of functions $\Phi^{(2)}(\tau)$ in bilogarithmic coordinates for the normal state of the cardiovascular system and a number of "catastrophic" arrhythmias (ventricular tachycardia, atrial fibrillation, atrial arrhythmia). An example is given of such a dependence for the state of the cardiovascular system—"ventricular tachycardia" (**Figure 11**) and atrial arrhythmia

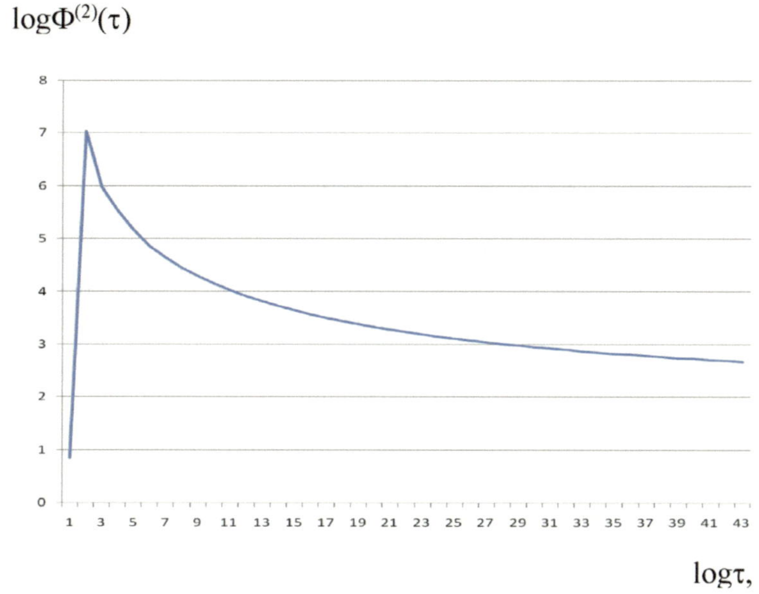

Figure 11.
Dependence $\log\Phi^{(2)}(\tau)$ for ventricular tachycardia.

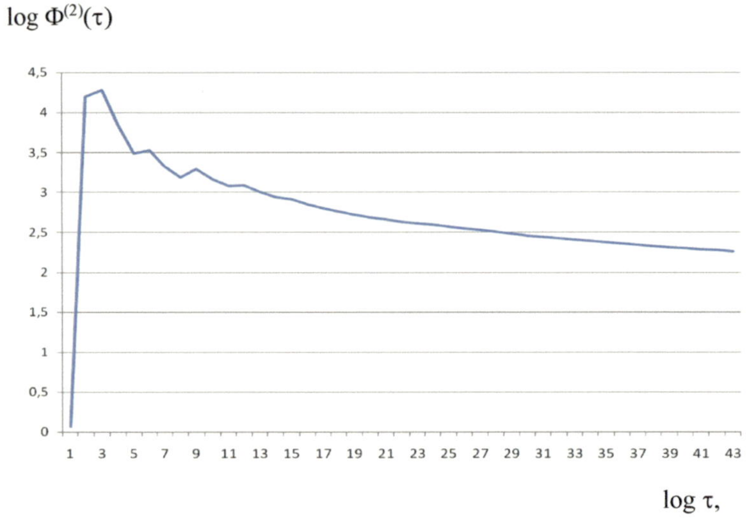

Figure 12.
Dependence $log\Phi^{(2)}(\tau)$ *for atrial rhythm.*

No.	ECG signal	σ_1	H_1	T_1
1	Norm	0.55	11.133	15.080
2	Atrial fibrillation	0.435	11.388	0.0640
3	Ventricular tachycardia	0.51	10.913	0.6840
4	Atrial arrhythmia	0.208	11.298	11.560

Table 2.
Informative parameters of the regular component.

(**Figure 12**). When conducting a computational experiment, we used the experimental data from the publicly available website www.PhysioNet.org.

For the considered conditions of the cardiovascular system, on the basis of the obtained dependencies, the informative parameters of the regular component of the ECG signals were calculated (**Table 2**).

Thus, for the considered functional conditions of the cardiovascular system, three informative parameters $n_0, T_0, S_s(0)$ for the singular component of the ECG signal and three informative diagnostic parameters σ_1, H_1, T_1 for the regular component of the ECG signal were obtained by flicker-noise spectroscopy.

A complex of six diagnostic parameters can be used to diagnose catastrophic conditions of the cardiovascular system (e.g., using an artificial neural network, where these parameters are considered as input data).

7. Fluctuation dynamics of electrocardiograms and the choice of sampling frequency of the studied signals

In the general case, when analyzing a complex chaotic signal measured at a certain sampling frequency f_d, a set of the indicated parameters is determined that characterizes the correlation interconnections in the sequences of irregularities-jumps and irregularities-bursts characteristic of a given signal determined with a sampling frequency of f_d. Thus, one of the main factors allowing to realize the allocation of the contribution of irregularities to the analyzed real signals is the

No.	ECG signal	Singular component			Regular component		
		$S_s(0)$	T_0	n_0	σ_1	H_1	T_1
1	Norm	437.80	0.0042	0.3414	0.55	11.133	15.080
2	Ventricular tachycardia	197.358	0.0032	0.4123	0.51	10.913	0.6840
3	Atrial fibrillation	334.364	0.0036	0.3836	0.435	11.388	0.0640
4	Atrial Arrhythmia	43.7105	0.0059	0.4013	0.208	11.298	11.560

Table 3.
Informative diagnostic parameters for various functional conditions of the cardiovascular system.

f_d, Hs	N	Singular component			Regular component			$\frac{4S(0)}{N}$
		$S_s(0)$	T_0	n_0	σ_1	H_1	T_1	
500	29.859	437.80	0.0042	0.3414	0.55	11.133	15.080	0.05
250	14.930	403.72	0.0028	0.4187	0.5044	10.845	1.38	0.08

Table 4.
Norm.

f_d, Hs	N	Singular component			Regular component			$\frac{4S(0)}{N}$
		$S_s(0)$	T_0	n	σ_1	H_1	T_1	
500	29.859	197.358	0.0032	0.4123	0.5180	10.913	0.6840	0.026
250	14.930	175.80	0.0034	0.3446	0.517	15.200	0.340	0.10

Table 5.
Ventricular tachycardia.

variation of the used frequencies f_d. If the analyzed time series is obtained at a sufficiently high sampling frequency f_d, then the analysis of dependencies $\Phi^{(2)}(\tau)$ and $S(f)$, calculated on the basis of time series obtained from the initial time series with a decreasing sampling frequency, allows us to estimate the measure of "stability" of parameters σ_1, T_1 and H_1 (for $\Phi^{(2)}(\tau)$) and the measure of variability of parameters $S_s(0), T_0$ and n_0 (for $S(f)$).

The high specificity of dependencies $\Phi^{(2)}(\tau)$ and $S(f)$ obtained by analyzing the state of complex systems can be used to diagnose diseases, as well as a combination of these parameters for their classification. We analyzed the four types of ECG signals—normal and cardiac "catastrophic" arrhythmias that directly threatened the patient's life, ventricular tachycardia, atrial fibrillation, and atrial arrhythmia. To identify the characteristics of the analyzed signals, it is necessary to evaluate the entire set of digitized data of $V(t)$ electrocardiograms for the indicated states of the cardiovascular system. When conducting the computational experiment, the experimental data from the public site www.PhysioNet.org were used.

The signals were taken from the II standard lead for ~60 s with a sampling frequency of f_d = 500 Hs and containing N = 29,859 values. Thus, a time series of ECG signals was obtained at a sufficiently high sampling frequency of f_d, since it can be used to obtain a set of new time series at sampling frequencies of less than f_d times.

The results of the corresponding analysis for the indicated functional conditions of the cardiovascular system at a sampling frequency of ECG signals f_d = 500 Hs are shown in **Table 3**.

We will carry out a comparative analysis of informative parameters for the two states of the cardiovascular system: normal (**Table 4**) and ventricular tachycardia (**Table 5**) for sampling frequencies f_d = 500 Hs and f_d = 250 Hs.

From the obtained tables, it follows that with increasing sampling frequency f_d, the high-frequency contribution to the power spectrum *S*(*f*) increases due to the inclusion of "bursts" in the analyzed signal corresponding to the increased frequency f_d. In this case, changes in dependence $\Phi^{(2)}(\tau)$ also occur at small τ, which are caused by the contribution of local changes in the values of the "laminar" signal sections. Therefore, with an increase of f_d, parameters T_0 and n_0, characterizing the high-frequency region of dependence *S*(*f*), and parameters H_1 and T_1, characterizing the dependence of $\Phi^{(2)}(\tau)$ for small τ, change. The value of parameter σ_1 and the nature of spectral dependence *S*(*f*) change to a much lesser extent. Small variations in the standard deviation parameter σ_1 indicate a smaller dependence of function $\Phi^{(2)}(\tau)$ on f_d. At the same time, the signal analysis in flicker-noise spectroscopy reveals the dynamics of changes in parameters H_1 and T_1 at small τ, as well as parameters T_0 andn_0, characterizing dependence *S*(*f*) in the high-frequency region. Since dependence *S*(*f*) is determined by the number of *M* terms in a discrete expression for *S*(*f*), it is convenient to use normalized expressions obtained by multiplying *S*(*f*) by a factor of $1/M = 4/N$ when changing the sampling frequencies. With this normalization, functional differences in dependence *S*(*f*), due to the use of signals measured at different sampling frequencies, are detected more explicitly.

Thus, when analyzing a complex chaotic signal during flicker-noise spectroscopy, a set of parameters is determined that characterize the correlation relationships in the sequences of irregularity-jumps and irregularity-bursts characteristic of this signal, determined with a sampling frequency of f_d. The analysis of dependencies $\Phi^{(2)}(\tau)$ and *S*(*f*), calculated on the basis of time series with decreasing sampling frequency, allows you to evaluate the measure of "stability" of parameters σ_1, T_1, and H_1, determined on the basis of $\Phi^{(2)}(\tau)$, and the measure of variability of the parameters $S_s(0), T_0$, and n_0, concerning dependence *S*(*f*).

8. The use of neural network technology in flicker-noise spectroscopy of an electrocardiogram

Based on a computational experiment, dependencies were obtained for the normal state of the cardiovascular system and a number of "catastrophic" arrhythmias (ventricular tachycardia, atrial fibrillation, atrial arrhythmia). We used the experimental data from the public website www.PhysioNet.org.

As a result of analyzing the power spectrum *S*(*f*), informative parameters were obtained for the singular component of the ECG signal: T_0, determining some characteristic time within which the measured dynamic variable is interconnected $V(t_i)$; n_0, dimensionless parameter that effectively determines how this relationship is lost as frequencies decrease to $1/2\pi T_0$; and $s(0)$, contribution to the power spectrum *S*(*f*), determined by the most high-frequency singular component [5].

The parameterization of the regular component of the ECG signal is carried out using expression $\Phi^{(2)}(\tau)$ with parameters T_1, τ_1, and H_1. In this case, parameter T_1 determines the characteristic time at which the values of the dynamic variables $V(t_i)$ do not correlate. To obtain reliable values of variance σ_1^2, it is necessary to calculate it at time intervals exceeding T_1. In this case, parameter H_1 shows by what law the relationship between the quantities $V(t_i)$ measured at different time instants is lost—the Hurst exponent.

Thus, when analyzing a complex chaotic signal, which is an ECG signal, we consider a set of six parameters, characterizing the correlation relationships in the sequences of irregularities—"jumps" and irregularities—"bursts" inherent in this signal.

9. The choice of artificial neural network and its characteristics

The obtained values of the parameters of the singular and regular component of the ECG signals can be used for differential diagnosis of the functional state of the cardiovascular system using artificial neural networks, where these parameters are considered as input data.

For the computational experiment, a perceptron three-layer network with direct connections was chosen (**Figure 13**).

To train the neural network, the backpropagation algorithm was used. The training time was about 240 s, the maximum network error was about 0.05, and the degree of training was about 0.01.

To recognize the pathologies of the cardiovascular system, a modular version of the structure of the construction of neural network blocks can be used (**Figure 14**).

The structure includes several parallel neural network modules, built on the basis of the structure of a multilayer perceptron. The advantage of this structure is the concentration of resources of each module on the recognition of only one pathology, which helps to reduce the likelihood of an error in the wrong conclusion for the whole system. In addition, the functionality of an artificial neural network is expanded by increasing the number of neural network modules to recognize new pathologies without retraining the entire system.

The main factor that allows one to distinguish the contribution of irregularities to the analyzed electrocardiographic signals is the variation of the used sampling frequencies f_d of the real signal. An analysis of the dependencies of the power spectrum and the second-order difference moment calculated on the basis of time series with a varying sampling frequency makes it possible to evaluate the measure of "stability" for the regular component and between the "variability" of its informative parameters for the singular component. In this case, parameter f_d can be used as an additional input parameter of an artificial neural network for recognition of the state of the cardiovascular system.

The presentation of electrocardiographic signals in the form of successive irregularities allows the use of flicker-noise spectroscopy in the analysis of such signals. The chaotic signal represented by the time series during flicker-noise spectroscopy allows one to parameterize these signals and determine informative diagnostic

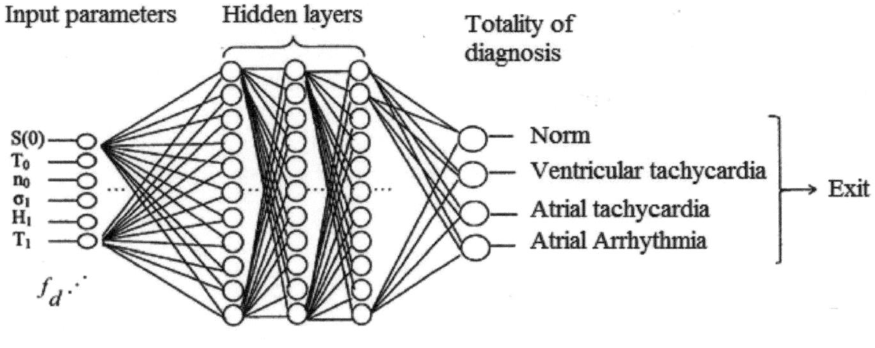

Figure 13.
The structural diagram of the proposed artificial neural network.

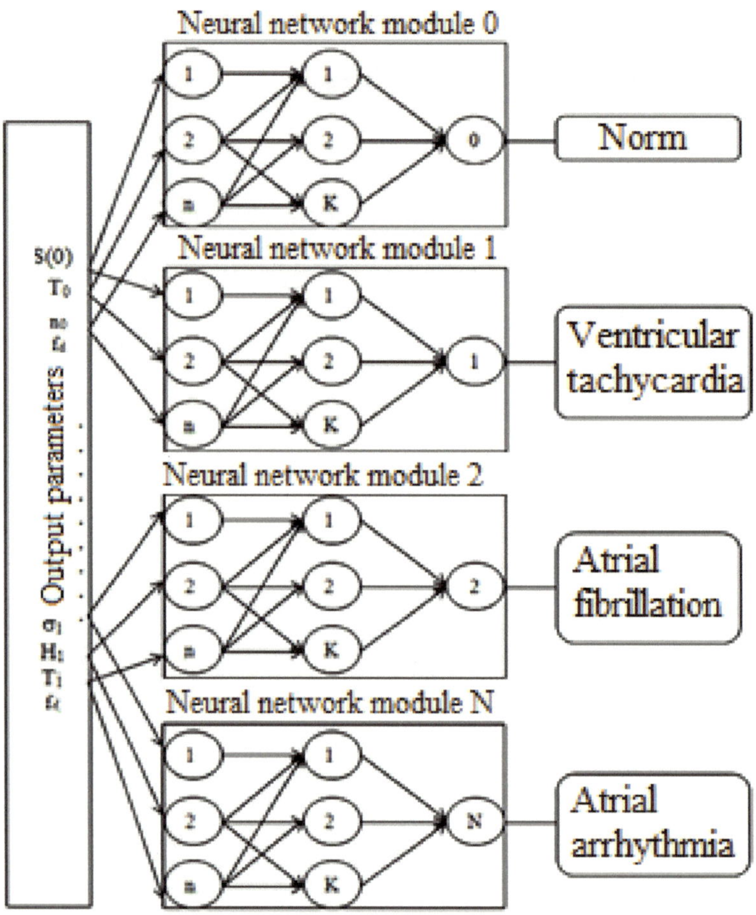

Figure 14.
A modular version of the construction of a neural network for recognition of pathologies (the number of input parameters, the number of neurons in the intermediate layer, the number of pathologies analyzed).

parameters, characterizing the functional state of the cardiovascular system. The set of informative parameters, as well as the sampling frequency of the signal, which determines the dynamics of changes in these parameters, allows the classification of heart diseases using a neural network.

Author details

Abdullayev Namiq Tahir* and Ahmadova Khadija Ramiz*
Department of Biomedical Engineering, Azerbaijan Technical University, Baku, Azerbaijan

*Address all correspondence to: a.namik46@mail.ru and phd.khadija@gmail.com

References

[1] Timashev SF. Flicker-Noise Spectroscopy: Information in Chaotic Signals. Moscow: FIZMATLIT; 2007. p. 248. (in Russia)

[2] Timashev SF, Polyakov YS. Review of flicker noise spectroscopy in electrochemistry. Fluctuation and Noise Letters. 2007;**7**(2):R15-R47

[3] Abdullaev NT, Dyshin OA, Gasankulieva MM. Flicker noise spectroscopy of electrocardiographic signals. Biomedical Engineering. 2016; **49**(5):268-273

[4] Abdullaev NT, Dyshin OA, Gasankulieva MM. Parameterization of the regular component of the ECG signal for diagnosis of the critical states of the cardiovascular system. Biomedical Engineering. 2016;**50**(3): 166-169

[5] Abdullaev NT, Gasankulieva MM, Dzhabieva ID. Application of neural network technology in flicker-noise spectroscopy of electrocardiograms. Information Technologies. 2018;**6**: 02-405 (in Russia)

Chapter 6

Biomedical Applications with Using Embedded Systems

Gulcicek Dere

Abstract

Besides the use of embedded systems in the field of electrical and electronics engineering, industrial, telecommunication, military, and many other commercial applications, and the other applications in the field of medical and biomedical are becoming increasingly common. Embedded system applications are increasing not only with designs on devices or with clothing, factories, medical and military equipments, portable devices, but also with applications such as 'mobile worlds' and 'e-worlds', Artificial Intelligence and IoT (Internet of things) with the possibility to make all kinds of software on them. In recent years, with the rise of infectious diseases such as the Covid 19 virus, there is a growing need for telemedicine applications such as diagnosis, prognosis and patient management. Embedded system technologies have occupied an important area in biomedical technology. Especially, to develop tools for the purposes of increasing the safety of healthcare workers in the event of epidemic infectious diseases in processes such as pandemics. For this purpose, monitoring of patients discharged from hospitals at home or non-intensive care beds during quarantine, or isolated in their homes, outpatient, and mildly ill, remotely, instantly, safely and quickly, are becoming increasingly important. In this section, we will give an overview of the embedded system structure and applications.

Keywords: biomedical applications, embedded systems, programmable device, biomedical hardware and software, medical devices

1. Introduction

Embedded systems are defined as customized hardware with an operating system and processor, designed to perform a specific operation alone. Systems consisting of a combination of software and hardware designed to enable a system consisting of mechanical and electronic components to work for a specific purpose through a microprocessor or microcontroller.

Embedded Systems usually do not interact directly with the end user. They work reactively and in real time with limited resources for a single purpose, and they can perform highly critical tasks from time to time in their usage areas.

Errors that may occur here can result in huge loss of property and lives. From this point of view, it is very important that these systems are "reliable" and "tolerant of errors".

Created by embedding software (hardware design for fpga) on a microcontroller, microprocessor, dsp (digital signal processor) or fpga (field programmable gate array); It is an electronic (or electromechanical) system that generally contains modules such as memory, input and output modules, sensors, physical output. It is an event that should not be confused with the dedicated system. Embedded systems that are generally smaller size and operate with smaller processor powers. Besides, the dedicated system is a system chosen to do a single work. For example, the library's web server and database server can be kept on separate machines, and if the task of these machines is to host only the web server, or only to provide the database, this is called a dedicated system. There is no size, processor or capacity constraint dedicated systems [1].

Is a programmable device, a combination of development hardware &software; that forms a component of an electrical device [2]. Medical applications of embedded systems are preferred because they are real-time and very fast. Embedded systems are computer systems and we need to know and control all the details and features of this computer system. An embedded system is a combination of both hardware and software, consisting of a microprocessor, memory for storing data and programs, converters microcontroller or digital signal processors (DSP), sensors, actuators and other interfaces [3].

2. Biomedical application of embedded systems

Embedded System Programming Tools can be listed as follows;

- Integrated Development Environments (IDE)
- Compiler
- Debug Devices and Software (Debugger)
- Emulators
- Testing Software and Devices
- Support Software

Embedded System Programming differs from other programming systems due to some features. Embedded software should use minimum program memory. Embedded software should not run slower than the system requires. It should be easy to interfere with embedded software and have high readability [4–12].

The most popular Embedded system medical applications are Imaging Devices. Although the working principles differ from each other, the common feature of imaging units such as MR, CT, PET (positron emission Tomography), US is that they are an embedded system.

Another example of medical applications of embedded systems is defibrillators. Defibrillators, a machine used to monitor a patient's heartbeat for an irregular pattern, and usually return the heartbeat to a normal pattern when an abnormal heartbeat is detected, are a useful example of biomedical applications of embedded systems.

Digital Flow sensors that monitor a patient's respiratory system, Blood pressure device and glucose test set, which is effective in detecting systolic and diastolic pressure of the human body, Fetal heart monitoring machine used during pregnancy, childbirth and childbirth to monitor the pulse of babies, device designs that allow users to monitor values such as heart rate, blood pressure, glucoses is an example of embedded systems.

It would not be wrong to say that there are computers in all devices. All into "embedded" computers there.

Small devices with embedded systems such as Raspberry pi, Ardunio can collect patient data and provide data processing with overwritten software, with the reduction in size and increase in processing power.

Similar small devices with embedded systems can make control decisions that can help provide better treatments and medications to patients.

Small designs with microcontrollers, sensors, motor drivers, sensors are also increasing. It provides practical and inexpensive solutions applied in case of any urgent need.

For example, studies such as 'the camera application that monitors social distance' has led us to better understand the importance of "social distance" that should exist between people, as it is transmitted by contact such as Covid19 and other infectious diseases. The progress, which has improved with vaccination studies all over the world, has now brought the quarantine process to an end and the return to social life. However, if the social distance is not maintained for infectious diseases, which are added every year, unfortunately, there will always be the risk of suffering from such diseases. Therefore, it is very important that we can maintain social distance in areas with high human density. For the solution of the problem, the first products used where practical solutions based on embedded system solutions such as smart phone application applications and smart wristband have been found practically.

Another solution to this problem is a software solutions via platform such as web API. But the disadvantage of these is their high cost. Thanks to the program overwritten using solutions such as NVIDIA, integrating the low-cost Intelligent Artificial Intelligence, Computer the existing cameras of the workplaces and providing real-time monitoring of social distance is another embedded system solution of the problem. Since it will be a product that can be mounted on existing cameras, there is no extra product expense other than the purchased kit.

Embedded system solutions offer fast, cheap and easily accessible solutions in other areas (**Figure 1**).

2.1 Embedded systems hardware

Embedded systems have already exceeded the limits of their name. Nowadays everything from smartphones to smart TVs, set top boxes to washing machines is actually an embedded system. They no longer have to perform certain tasks, they can do many tasks at the same time.

They are electronic systems designed to perform a certain function, microprocessors are used for the central processing unit in systems with low processing load (fire alarm, etc.), while in systems we call hard-real time (systems that will result in the transition from life to death at the smallest delay), micro-processors are used for

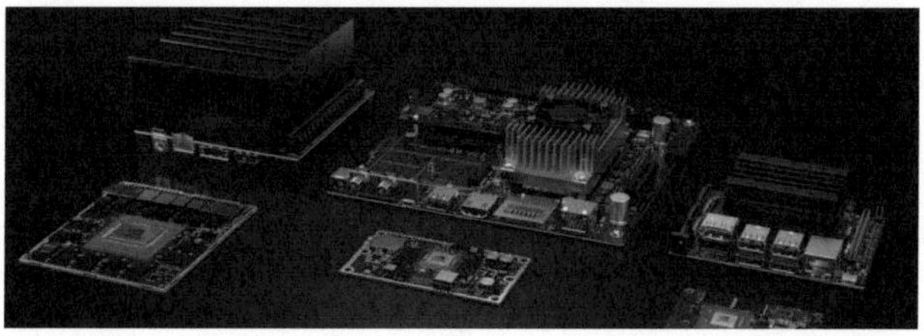

Figure 1.
NVIDIA Jetson solutions [8].

the central processing unit. Systems used for reading sensors such as temperature, humidity, gas, flow, ultrasonic. B, etc. are also embedded systems. This world can be stepped into with affordable and easy-to-use embedded systems (Arduino) for hobbyists.

Embedded systems are systems that host low power processors within high frequency processors, have an operating system or direct, real-time management infrastructure within their related processes, and provide control of sensors and trainers. Although the volume of transactions generally remains lower than computer systems, it has started to close this gap in the development of today's technology and industry 4.0 studies. Embedded system design takes up a lot of space at the point of performing operations-based activities such as rationalizing robotic systems, artificial intelligence and machine learning.

Survey studies have shown that the most important software/hardware tools are, respectively; Oscilloscope, Debugger, Compiler/assembler, IDE, Logic analyzer, JTAG/BDM, Software libraries, Linux tools, ICE, Configuration Management tools, Static Analysis tools, Software drivers etc. It is necessary to know very well about digital electronics hardware. The devices studied have been created with logic gates and every subject of digital electronics, every basic circuit is located on microcontrollers and digital devices. Since the devices used are not simple devices, it is not possible to understand them with half information.

Embedded systems are computer systems and it is necessary to know and control all the details and features of this computer system. We see that many of them are indexed to a hardware and describe embedded systems through that hardware.

Hardware components are basically as follows;

- MCU (MicroController Unit), FPGA, ASIC etc.
- General purpose input–output units (GPIO)
- Communication units
- System-specific components

Microcontrollers, one of the basic parts of embedded systems, can be defined as a single chip computer. They contain a microprocessor, memory, digital inputs-outputs and other peripherals (timer, interrupt, ADC etc.). Some of well known microcontrollers are; RX Family, RL78, 78 K, H8 Family, V850, RH850, STM8, STM32, RA, Synergy, RE R8C.

Advanced embedded systems as it may seem there is no need for an analog electronic information. Basic and practical electronic knowledge can be sufficient.

The software parts are basically collected under 3 main headings; Real time operating system (RTOS), Third party software libraries and Software applications.

A table about the boards used in the design of the embedded system, included in the survey conducted by the Aspencore group in 2017, is below (**Table 1**).

There are indispensable Measuring Instruments for embedded system laboratories in both Biomedical and other fields. These are for example; Digital Oscilloscope, Function Generator, Tabletop Digital Multimeter, Power Supply, Computer, Projector etc. Depending on the design work and studied, needed help tools and measuring instruments varies. For example, while working with **Arduino**, which is a simplified framework designed for artists and designers who are not very interested in electronics and computer science, the measuring instruments needed and those working with sensors may differ (**Figure 2**).

Development Board Started With (Write-in Answers Only)	N = 356	Percent
ST Microelectronics	38	10.7%
TI (LaunchPad = 5)	38	10.7%
Xilinx	29	8.1%
NXP	26	7.3%
Microchip	21	5.9%
Arduino	20	5.6%
Rasberry Pi	15	4.2%
BeagleBoard Bone Black	12	3.4%
Atmel	10	2.8%
Freescale (NXP)	10	2.8%
Cypress kits	6	1.7%
Renasas	6	1.7%
Altera Stratix V DSP Kit	5	1.4%
Avnet	5	1.4%
Intel Edison	5	1.4%
Silicon Labs	4	1.1%
Digi	3	0.8%
ESP32	3	0.8%
MSP430 – TI	3	0.8%
Nordic/nRF52-DK	3	0.8%

Table 1.
Answers to the question of "Did you start your current embedded design with a development board?" in Aspencore 2017 survey [13].

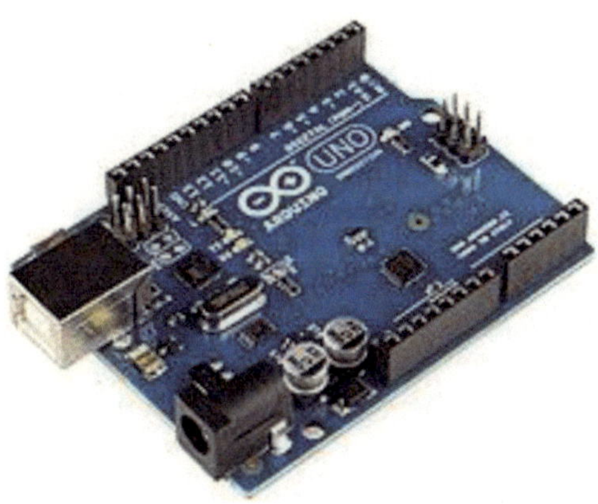

Figure 2.
Arduino Uno SMD R3 [14].

The main factor in Arduino spreading this much is the software part. The Integrated Development Environment (**IDE**) required to develop software on Arduino can be downloaded free from the website. It can be developed easily with the development environment that can run on Windows, Mac and Linux platforms.

The Arduino IDE is based on a programming language called Processing and a project called Wiring. In the development environment, which is very easy to use, you can easily compile Arduino programs (called sketch) and upload them to your card. A language similar to C ++ is used as the programming language. Thanks to the existing libraries, many operations and communication between peripherals can be performed easily. One of the Arduino's most powerful features is that it has an extensible library system. Thus, libraries written for new peripherals can be easily integrated.

One of the most beautiful features of the Arduino is that new hardware features can be added with additional cards called "shield". Thanks to these additional cards that are compatible with the Arduino board, it is possible to realize many different projects. Examples of these attachments are modules such as Bluetooth, wifi, motor driver, LCD screen.

Sensors, which are another hardware in embedded systems, are designed that can serve many different purposes with the developing technology. These are advanced technology embedded sensor systems such as MEMS/NEMS and optical technologies to be used in Internet applications of objects, Sensors resistant to extreme conditions, Sensors with innovative features (according to which high sensitivity and resolution, cost effective, reliable (robust), Self-calibrating; resistant to errors, losses, deterioration), Intelligent sensor technologies that can be used in the production process, Packaged, long-lasting, directly connected to the cloud, capable of running multiple applications, expandable, easily configurable sensors and components.

2.2 Embedded systems software

Electronics about to have a lot of information, even to design eye fabulous indoor circuit cards unless you know the computer science genius, will not be a nice software in embedded systems. In fact, the software is now being used for other circuits in embedded system control software. Applications such as image processing, web server, user interface, operating system are now also written for embedded systems.

While working on embedded systems will need to use a high percentage of the C language. Although languages such as Java and C ++ are used in some different areas, and the Assembly is used in applications of hardware that require performance or that do not have a C compiler, generally no language other than C is used. The results of the embedded systems market research conducted by the Aspencore group in 2017, the survey conducted with companies and engineers working in the field of embedded systems showed that the most used languages (**Figure 3**);

The C language is the most preferred because it has both medium and high-level features, increases efficiency by producing less code, is quite common in embedded software libraries, is very well-known, is a compiler for almost all microcontrollers, and access to resources is high.

The most used operating systems in embedded systems are; Embedded Linux, FreeRTOS, In-house/custom, Android, Debian (Linux), Ubuntu, Microsoft (Windows Embedded 7 / Standard), Texas Instruments RTOS, Texas Instruments (DSP/BIOS), Micrium (uC/OS-III), Microsoft (Windows 7 Compact or earlier...), and also Integrity, OSE, SCIOPTA, seL4, Pharos, FreeRTOS, QNX.

Embedded system development is also changing rapidly. While working with microcontrollers with small-sized resources in the past, it is possible to talk about products that reach very high speeds today. Nowadays, subjects such as internet protocols and encryption algorithms appear as new study areas. Naturally, it is

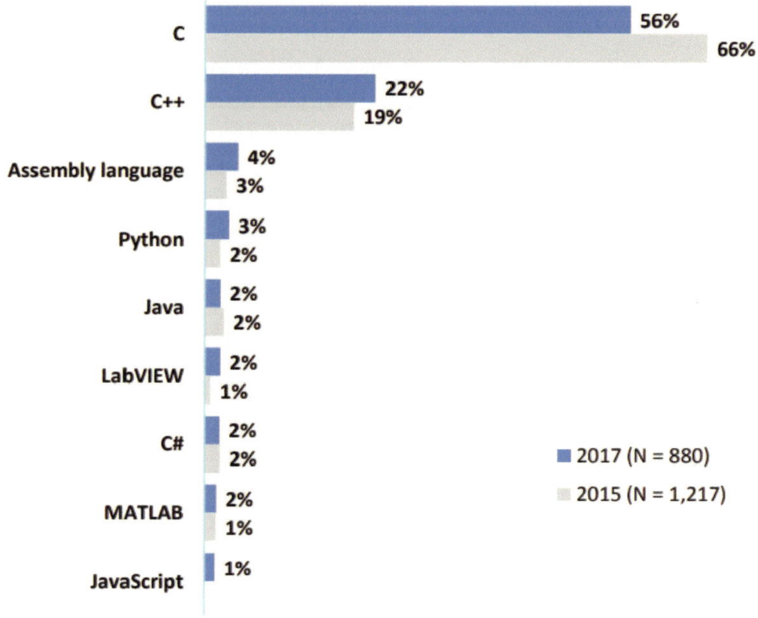

Figure 3.
Answers to the question of "My current embedded project is programmed mostly in" in Aspencore 2017 survey [13].

becoming a necessity to use ready-made modules on the platforms we work with. As programming becomes increasingly complex, we now need platforms that support us. The structure known as Internet of Things (**IOT**) has modules called "gateways" that will connect other modules and devices to the network.

With the development of new generation communication infrastructure and standards, it is ensured that high value added, user-friendly service, analysis, monitoring, decision-making and control applications are developed by developing equipment that can work with new generation protocol structures and also adapt to standard protocols.

At the same time, these IOT structures have implemented and comply with the standards required to develop manageable, controllable and secure system architectures, to communicate safely with the sensor, to have a high level of service in order not to cause a disruption in production, to support local and foreign standards, to work openly with different platforms when necessary, to have programming intermediates for different applications, to have a scalable and traceable structure, to perform system health monitoring of end units and platform components when necessary must be able to work in all kinds of environments and operating systems (mobile, etc.).

Another attractive point in embedded system software is coding. The minimum area, minimum time, writing is the most appropriate considering the principle of maximum benefit. It is the most appropriate to write with the principle of minimum space, minimum time and maximum benefit.

2.3 Medical device design

Medical device technology, one of the most practical field of embedded hardware and software technology. In addition to the previously mentioned medical imaging systems, Biomedical power units, Clinical and Biotechnological Analyzers, Portable Diagnostic Systems, Mobile Patient Monitoring Systems, Nurse Call

Systems, Patient Queue Systems and their designs are also made with embedded system applications.

Apart from academic studies, there is also a large business area in the biomedical field. These medical embedded systems, embedded computing or customer needs for projects should be ready for SBC (Single Board Computer) use. They offer high performance and low cost effective solutions to entrepreneurs, medical staff and patients in the medical sector. Low-power and high-performance portable embedded systems offer many diagnostic functions, save time, aim to reduce overall diagnostic costs.

There is another card that is frequently used in electronic, robotic and biomedical designs like Arduino, it is Raspberry Pi. Arduino does not have an operating system. It can only run programs compiled for the Arduino platform, which means programs, mostly written in C ++. Raspberry Pi usually runs an operating system that is Linux. In other words, it can be called a mini computer with this feature. The Raspberry Pi is the smallest computer. They look quite similar at first glance. Pins, connectors, screw holes etc. In fact, both cards are very, very different from each other. The fact that the ram and microprocessors are much larger makes the Raspberry pi stand out in terms of software. It is an alternative portable computer especially image processing applications in biomedical studies (**Figure 4**).

Medical devices that can perform image processing and many other operations are developed especially with software such as opencv simplecv. For example, working on an image taken with a medical modality is also possible with embedded system solutions. You can perform the software you make on a normal computer on image processing with an embedded system tool such as raspberry pi, arduino, nvidia or a more advanced mini computer or cards. For example, you can perform image processing such as edge detection over the image, thanks to the related software you wrote on the Raspberry pi and a monitor connected to it [16–19].

2.4 Embedded systems restrictions

When coding on an embedded system, it is necessary to pay attention to the detail between optimization and readability of the code. If there is enough memory, a readable code may be preferred instead of optimization. Many certification processes are required for the newly developed product (IEC 62304, EN 50128,

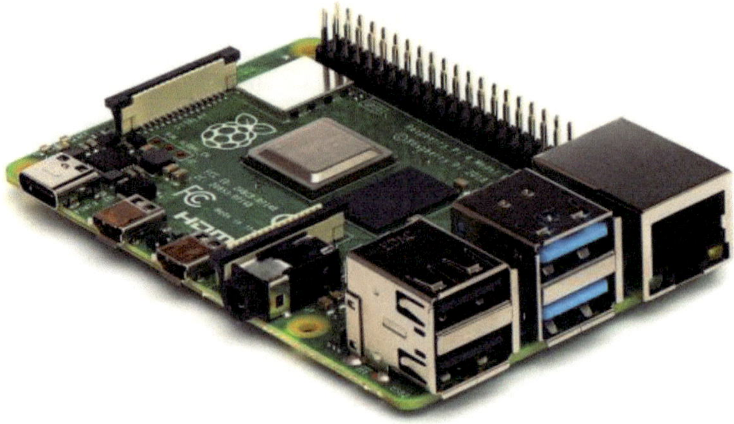

Figure 4.
Raspberry pi 4 model B [15].

EN 50657, ISO 26262, IEC 61508 etc.). IEC 62304 is an important international standard, especially for medical devices. But a simple PCBs certificate cost can thousands of dollars [16–19].

To calibrate an analog sensor, it is necessary to communicate with the software via SPI and I2C. If such a digital sensor is not controlled by software, the operation is not successful. The problems that cause problems in the process of embedded system design are listed as follows; Debugging tools, Schedule, engineering team skill level, firmware itself, microprocessor, programming tools, interfaces, other hardware.

Restrictions are basically;

- Cost
- Processing power
- Memory
- Power consumption

Additionally, hardware vulnerability situations such as Meltdown and Specter, caused by a hardware deficit in processors, are also a problem for embedded system solutions.

3. Conclusions

Current and developing features show that embedded system applications will increasingly continue to be used in biomedical applications, as in all areas of use.

Expectation from embedded system application in biomedical systems as in others; industrial endpoint devices with various sensors on them are fault-tolerant and self-calibrated systems that aim to be able to influence the outside world and generate meaningful data, have a process capability when necessary, have a logical and virtual sensor approach. It is inevitable that the number of companies designing embedded systems will increase and the market will grow. New and better versions of the design cards are expected to be launched. The increase in software libraries and the low cost of embedded systems in health care will cause them to be preferred more because of their portability. It is also predicted that artificial intelligence applications in health will continue to increase with systems integrated with embedded systems and new software.

Any other expectations;

- Monitoring of vital health parameters (sleep, epilepsy, heart, etc.), recording, wireless transfer and digital transfer (phone, tablet, computer, etc.)
- Wearable devices; Flexible electronic devices capable of energy harvesting and storage, technologies that can send data to the cloud and receive commands, and can be worn compatible with the Internet of Things
- Sensors and devices that increase portability
- Protective personal-real-time in vivo measurement systems
- Having e-health software that can run on common platforms

- Tele-radiology, tele-rehabilitation
- Systems for the development of preventive and preventive health services and personalized medical monitoring systems
- Computer-cloud interfaces
- Biosignal acquisition and processing
- Virtual reality systems and 3D training and treatment simulators
- Network based devices
- ICT Based Innovative Medical Devices

Apart from these, it is not difficult to predict that new designs will be made in line with the needs that have not yet come to mind.

The applications of embedded systems, which are generally tried to be explained in more basic lines, make them more preferable due to the increasing need arising and their practical and low cost. Embedded system applications where real-time solutions, ANN, CNN, Machine Learning, Deep Learning, Federated Learning, NLP applications and more are used together or separately will increase in diversity.

Author details

Gulcicek Dere
Yeditepe University, Istanbul, Turkey

*Address all correspondence to: gulcicekdere@yahoo.com

References

[1] "Embedded systems medical and biomedical applications." December 2020. Retrieved from https://microcontrollerslab.com/embedded-systems-medical-applications/

[2] Carolo, Lucas. "Arduino vs Raspberry Pi: The Differences". All3DP. December, 2020. https://all3dp.com/2/arduino-vs-raspberry-pi/

[3] Copes, Flavio "Arduino vs Raspberry Pi; A comparison of two of the most popular platforms to tinker with", February 2019. Retrieved from https://flaviocopes.com/arduino-vs-raspberry-pi/

[4] Tyler Ross Lambert. "Introduction to Microcontrollers and Embedded Systems". Auburn University. July 2017.

[5] Embedded Staff. "2017 Embedded Markets Study; Integrating IoT and Advanced Technology Designs, Application Development & Processing Environments", Aspencore, April 2017.

[6] Panneerselvam, Priya. "Embedded System in Biomedical Applications: Challenges Ahead". International Journal of Science, Engineering and Technology Research, Volume 3, Issue 9, September 2014.

[7] Frank Vahid, Tony Givargis. "Embedded System Design: A Unified Hardware/Software Introduction". Wiley; New edition. October, 2001. ISBN-10: 0471386782

[8] NVIDIA Web Site, Retrieved from January 2021. https://www.nvidia.com/tr-tr/autonomous-machines/jetson-store/

[9] Clarke, Peter (2000-07-28). "STMicroelectronics buys WaferScale Integration" *EE Times*. Retrieved 2020-12-09.

[10] Wikipedia. 'RISC-V. January 2021. Retrieved from https://en.wikipedia.org/wiki/Raspberry_Pi

[11] "Procedure Call Standard for the ARM Architecture" (PDF). Arm Holdings. Retrieved 27 May 2013.

[12] "Some facts about the Acorn RISC Machine" Roger Wilson posting to comp.arch, Retrieved 25 May 2007.

[13] Demir, Asim Ahmed, "Gömülü Sistemler ve Gömülü Sistemlerde Yazılım Tasarımı" , EMO Ankara, January 2019.

[14] Wikipedia. "Arduino". December, 2020. Retrieved from https://en.wikipedia.org/wiki/Arduino

[15] Wikipedia. "Raspberry Pi". December, 2020. Retrieved from https://en.wikipedia.org/wiki/Raspberry_Pi

[16] Manikandan L C et all., Hardware implementation of fast bilateral filter and canny edge detector using Raspberry Pi for telemedicine applications, March 2020. Journal of Ambient Intelligence and Humanized Computing

[17] Dere Gulcicek, Fetal Length Calculation Utilizing Edge Detection Method on Raspberry Pi 3, 21st National Biomedical Engineering Meeting (BIYOMUT), 2017

[18] Vilem Srovnal et all., "Embedded System Design for Health Supervisory Systems", Ubiquitous Computing and Communication Journal, 2010.

[19] Fabio Rossi et all., "Embedded Bio-Mimetic System for Functional Electrical Stimulation Controlled by Event-Driven sEMG", Applications in Electronics Pervading Industry, Environment and Society – Sensing Systems and Pervasive Intelligence, 2020.